FAST FACTS for
the **HOSPICE NURSE**

D1118367

OTHER FAST FACTS BOOKS

Fast Facts for the NEW NURSE PRACTITIONER: What You Really Need to Know in a Nutshell, 2e (*Aktan*)

Fast Facts for the ER NURSE: Emergency Room Orientation in a Nutshell, 2e (*Buettner*)

Fast Facts About GI AND LIVER DISEASES FOR NURSES: What APRNs Need to Know in a Nutshell (*Chaney*)

Fast Facts for the MEDICAL–SURGICAL NURSE: Clinical Orientation in a Nutshell (*Ciocco*)

Fast Facts for the NURSE PRECEPTOR: Keys to Providing a Successful Preceptorship in a Nutshell (*Ciocco*)

Fast Facts for the OPERATING ROOM NURSE: An Orientation and Care Guide in a Nutshell (*Criscitelli*)

Fast Facts for the ANTEPARTUM AND POSTPARTUM NURSE: A Nursing Orientation and Care Guide in a Nutshell (*Davidson*)

Fast Facts for the NEONATAL NURSE: A Nursing Orientation and Care Guide in a Nutshell (*Davidson*)

Fast Facts About PRESSURE ULCER CARE FOR NURSES: How to Prevent, Detect, and Resolve Them in a Nutshell (*Dziedzic*)

Fast Facts for the GERONTOLOGY NURSE: A Nursing Care Guide in a Nutshell (*Eliopoulos*)

Fast Facts for the LONG-TERM CARE NURSE: What Nursing Home and Assisted Living Nurses Need to Know in a Nutshell (*Eliopoulos*)

Fast Facts for the CLINICAL NURSE MANAGER: Managing a Changing Workplace in a Nutshell, 2e (*Fry*)

Fast Facts for EVIDENCE-BASED PRACTICE: Implementing EBP in a Nutshell, 2e (*Godshall*)

Fast Facts About NURSING AND THE LAW: Law for Nurses in a Nutshell (*Grant, Ballard*)

Fast Facts for the L&D NURSE: Labor & Delivery Orientation in a Nutshell, 2e (*Groll*)

Fast Facts for the RADIOLOGY NURSE: An Orientation and Nursing Care Guide in a Nutshell (*Grossman*)

Fast Facts on ADOLESCENT HEALTH FOR NURSING AND HEALTH PROFESSIONALS: A Care Guide in a Nutshell (*Herrman*)

Fast Facts for the FAITH COMMUNITY NURSE: Implementing FCN/Parish Nursing in a Nutshell (*Hickman*)

Fast Facts for the CARDIAC SURGERY NURSE: Caring for Cardiac Surgery Patients in a Nutshell, 2e (*Hodge*)

Fast Facts for the CLINICAL NURSING INSTRUCTOR: Clinical Teaching in a Nutshell, 2e (*Kan, Stabler-Haas*)

Fast Facts for the WOUND CARE NURSE: Practical Wound ~~Management in a Nutshell (Kifer)~~

Fast Facts About EKGs FOR NURSES: The Rules of ~~Identifying~~

Fast Facts for the CRITICAL CARE NURSE: Critical Care ~~N~~

D1043148

Fast Facts for the TRAVEL NURSE: Travel Nursing in a Nutshell (*Landrum*)

Fast Facts for the SCHOOL NURSE: School Nursing in a Nutshell, 2e (*Loschiavo*)

Fast Facts About CURRICULUM DEVELOPMENT IN NURSING: How to Develop & Evaluate Educational Programs in a Nutshell (*McCoy, Anema*)

Fast Facts for DEMENTIA CARE: What Nurses Need to Know in a Nutshell (*Miller*)

Fast Facts for HEALTH PROMOTION IN NURSING: Promoting Wellness in a Nutshell (*Miller*)

Fast Facts for STROKE CARE NURSING: An Expert Guide in a Nutshell (*Morrison*)

Fast Facts for the MEDICAL OFFICE NURSE: What You Really Need to Know in a Nutshell (*Richmeier*)

Fast Facts for the PEDIATRIC NURSE: An Orientation Guide in a Nutshell (*Rupert, Young*)

Fast Facts About the GYNECOLOGICAL EXAM FOR NURSE PRACTITIONERS: Conducting the GYN Exam in a Nutshell (*Secor, Fantasia*)

Fast Facts for the STUDENT NURSE: Nursing Student Success in a Nutshell (*Stabler-Haas*)

Fast Facts for CAREER SUCCESS IN NURSING: Making the Most of Mentoring in a Nutshell (*Vance*)

Fast Facts for the TRIAGE NURSE: An Orientation and Care Guide in a Nutshell (*Visser, Montejano, Grossman*)

Fast Facts for DEVELOPING A NURSING ACADEMIC PORTFOLIO: What You Really Need to Know in a Nutshell (*Wittmann-Price*)

Fast Facts for the HOSPICE NURSE: A Concise Guide to End-of-Life Care (*Wright*)

Fast Facts for the CLASSROOM NURSING INSTRUCTOR: Classroom Teaching in a Nutshell (*Yoder-Wise, Kowalski*)

Forthcoming FAST FACTS Books

Fast Facts About PTSD: A Clinician's Guide to Post-Traumatic Stress Disorder in a Nutshell (*Adams*)

Fast Facts for Nurses About PARKINSON'S DISEASE: An Expert Guide in a Nutshell (*Armitage*)

Fast Facts for the ER NURSE: Emergency Department Orientation in a Nutshell, 3e (*Buettner*)

Fast Facts on COMBATING NURSE BULLYING, INCIVILITY, AND WORKPLACE VIOLENCE: What Nurses Need to Know in a Nutshell (*Ciocco*)

Fast Facts for TESTING AND EVALUATION IN NURSING: Teaching Skills in a Nutshell (*Dusaj*)

Fast Facts for Nurses About HOME INFUSION THERAPY: The Expert's Best Practice Guide in a Nutshell (*Gorski*)

Fast Facts About the NURSING PROFESSION: Historical Perspectives in a Nutshell (*Hunt*)

Fast Facts for the CLINICAL NURSING INSTRUCTOR: Nursing Student Success in a Nutshell, 3e (*Kan, Stabler-Haas*)

Fast Facts for the CRITICAL CARE NURSE: Critical Care Nursing in Nutshell, 2e (*Landrum*)

Fast Facts About NURSING PATIENTS WITH MENTAL ILLNESS (MI): What RNs, NPs, and New Psych Nurses Need to Know (*Marshall*)

Fast Facts About the GYNECOLOGIC EXAM: A Professional Guide for NPs, PAs, and Midwives, 2e (*Secor, Fantasia*)

Patricia Moyle Wright, PhD, CRNP, CNS, CHPN, CNE, has worked in hospice and palliative care for more than 20 years, beginning as a nursing assistant, later as a registered nurse, and now as a family nurse practitioner. She earned bachelor's and master's degrees in nursing from Misericordia University, Dallas, Pennsylvania, and a PhD in nursing from Loyola University, Chicago, Illinois. Dr. Wright is a board-certified adult health clinical nurse specialist and family nurse practitioner. She is also a certified hospice and palliative nurse (CHPN) and a certified nurse educator (CNE).

Dr. Wright is an associate professor in the department of nursing at The University of Scranton. She teaches a number of graduate and undergraduate courses, including a course on end-of-life care. Dr. Wright has published numerous articles and book chapters on end-of-life issues, including grief and bereavement. Her most recent work is a coedited book, *Perinatal and Pediatric Bereavement in Nursing and Other Health Professions* (Springer Publishing), winner of an American Journal of Nursing Book of the Year Award.

FAST FACTS for the **HOSPICE NURSE**

A Concise Guide to End-of-Life Care

Patricia Moyle Wright, PhD, CRNP, CNS, CHPN, CNE

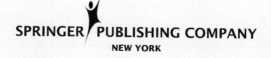

SPRINGER PUBLISHING COMPANY
NEW YORK

Springer Publishing Company, LLC
11 West 42nd Street
New York, NY 10036
www.springerpub.com

Acquisitions Editor: Elizabeth Nieginski
Senior Production Editor: Kris Parrish
Composition: Westchester Publishing Services

ISBN: 978-0-8261-3198-0
e-book ISBN: 978-0-8261-3199-7

17 18 19 20 21 / 5 4 3 2 1

The author and the publisher of this Work have made every effort to use sources believed to be reliable to provide information that is accurate and compatible with the standards generally accepted at the time of publication. Because medical science is continually advancing, our knowledge base continues to expand. Therefore, as new information becomes available, changes in procedures become necessary. We recommend that the reader always consult current research and specific institutional policies before performing any clinical procedure. The author and publisher shall not be liable for any special, consequential, or exemplary damages resulting, in whole or in part, from the readers' use of, or reliance on, the information contained in this book. The publisher has no responsibility for the persistence or accuracy of URLs for external or third-party Internet websites referred to in this publication and does not guarantee that any content on such websites is, or will remain, accurate or appropriate.

Library of Congress Cataloging-in-Publication Data

Title: Fast facts for the hospice nurse : a concise guide to end-of-life care / Patricia Moyle Wright.
Other titles: Fast facts (Springer Publishing Company)
Description: New York, NY : Springer Publishing Company, LLC, [2017] | Series: Fast facts | Includes bibliographical references.
Identifiers: LCCN 2016055477 (print) | LCCN 2016056007 (ebook) | ISBN 9780826131980 (hard copy) | ISBN 9780826131997 (ebook)
Subjects: | MESH: Hospice Care | Hospice and Palliative Care Nursing | Nurse's Role
Classification: LCC RT87.T45 (print) | LCC RT87.T45 (ebook) | NLM WY 152.3 | DDC 616.02/9—dc23
LC record available at https://lccn.loc.gov/2016055477

Contact us to receive discount rates on bulk purchases.
We can also customize our books to meet your needs.
For more information please contact: sales@springerpub.com

Printed in the United States of America by Gasch Printing.

This book is lovingly dedicated to the memory of all of the hospice patients who allowed me to care for them during their most sacred and vulnerable hours.

Contents

Foreword

I began working in hospice care in 1980 when the field was in its infancy. There were few resources for nurses. Most people could not pronounce the word "hospice" and few had any idea of what it meant. Much has changed since that time and, fortunately, hospice has steadily evolved to become the gold standard of high-quality, patient-centered, compassionate care. It is now a familiar word and, more importantly, we now have generations of families who have come to know hospice because hospices have cared for those they love.

There are, however, some things that remain unchanged. Today, as in 1980, there remains an urgent need for practical resources to guide the daily practice of hospice nurses. Dr. Patricia Moyle Wright, editor of the beautiful text *Perinatal and Pediatric Bereavement*, has created another great resource for nurses through this book on hospice. The content of this book takes us back to our roots in hospice, with content on hospice philosophy, real "nuts and bolts" on hospice requirements, and a concise summary of often-neglected topics, such as existential suffering, cultural concerns, and quality assurance. The book also addresses the important topic of self-care. This is a book for the busy hospice nurse who has great compassion but limited time.

Betty Ferrell, PhD, MA, RN, FAAN, FPCN, CHNP
Professor and Director
Nursing Research
City of Hope Medical Center
Duarte, California

Preface

Every nurse cares for a patient facing end-of-life issues at some point in his or her career, sometimes when it is least expected. *Fast Facts for the Hospice Nurse: A Concise Guide to End-of-Life Care* is intended to be a valuable, up-to-date resource for nurses who provide end-of-life care in hospice, long-term care, or even acute care settings. This book is for nurses who are seeking to specialize in hospice, as well as for those who are seeking to enhance their knowledge of end-of-life care within other specialties. Each part of the book addresses topics that help orient the nurse to hospice philosophy and approaches to end-of-life care. Numerous resources are provided throughout the book, and "Fast Facts in a Nutshell" boxes highlight important pieces of information. Each part of the book is designed to provide nurses with a concise overview of another facet of end-of-life care.

, Part I differentiates hospice from palliative care. Hospice care is presented as a specialized area of nursing practice, which incorporates aspects of palliative care, but also has unique features. Also in this part, a timeline is provided, tracing the hospice movement and highlighting the various social and legislative changes that supported the growth of hospice care in the United States. As hospice became a recognized specialty, the scope and standards of practice were delineated, and specialty certification became an option. Part I closes with an overview of the specific role of the registered nurse within the hospice interdisciplinary team.

In Part II, the "nuts and bolts" of hospice nursing are reviewed. Advanced skills, such as discussing end-of-life wishes and documenting patients' wishes in an advanced care plan, are discussed. Hospice admission criteria are also presented. Using these criteria, nurses can have a powerful impact by identifying patients who might benefit from hospice care. When a patient is medically appropriate for hospice and chooses to forgo curative treatment, a hospice admission can take place. This part closes with an overview of the hospice admission process and how to determine the appropriate level of hospice care for each patient.

Part III covers crucial aspects of direct end-of-life nursing care, with a focus on spiritual and physical suffering. An overview of several major world religions, including Buddhism, Christianity, Hinduism, Islam, and Judaism, is provided with information on common religiously based end-of-life preferences. Additionally, this part provides information on how to assess and respond to various physical symptoms that are common at the end of life. These include anxiety, edema, constipation, delirium, dyspnea, nausea and vomiting, pain, and terminal secretions.

Also in Part III is a discussion of how to help caregivers and family members identify signs of approaching death and how to provide support throughout the dying process. Current understandings of grief and bereavement theories provide a foundation for nurses to assess families' responses to the loss of a loved one, identify "red flags," and implement effective interventions with the interdisciplinary team.

In Part IV, the emphasis shifts from providing direct patient and family care to ensuring consistent delivery and documentation of quality care. An overview of the development of guidelines for hospice and palliative care is provided, along with a discussion of how these clinical guidelines led to the development of quality indicators. Therefore, quality reporting, which was at one time voluntary, is now mandatory for full reimbursement from Medicare. Quality reporting requirements for Medicare reimbursement, as well as quality indicators that may be useful for internal benchmarking, are reviewed. Use of the electronic health record, including its usefulness in ensuring that documentation includes vital information for regulators, and internal quality monitoring initiatives are also discussed.

Part V, the final part of the book, focuses on the often-overlooked, but extremely important topic of self-care. In this part, sources of job stress for hospice nurses are noted, with a particular emphasis on interpersonal issues such as lateral violence, generational differences in the workplace, and personality types. The consequences of job stress on individuals and organizations are discussed, followed by recommendations for addressing job stress. This part ends with an overview of how to navigate a toxic workplace and how to utilize various self-care techniques.

Fast Facts for the Hospice Nurse is a vital resource for nurses who work with patients facing terminal illness. This portable guide is packed with information regarding the growth of hospice in the United States, hospice certification, criteria for hospice admission, levels of care in hospice, working with the hospice interdisciplinary team, recommendations for the nursing care of hospice patients and families, and treatment options for common end-of-life symptoms. A unique feature of this book is the special emphasis on job stress in hospice nursing, working in a toxic environment, and the use of self-care techniques for health care professionals. This book is a critical resource for anyone who wishes to learn more about caring for patients and families facing end-of-life issues.

Patricia Moyle Wright

Acknowledgments

I gratefully acknowledge the love and support of my family, particularly my parents, who taught me to do work that has meaning and helps others. I also gratefully acknowledge the hard work and support of my in-house editors, David and Dominic, and the encouragement of my personal cheerleader, Vivian.

I am grateful for the support of my hospice colleagues, some of whom have been my friends for more than 20 years. They are a source of inspiration for me. In particular, I wish to acknowledge Judith Spitale, MSN, RN, who gave me my first hospice job as a nursing assistant and has been a steadfast role model for many years.

Special acknowledgement is due to Elizabeth Nieginski and Rachel Landes, editors at Springer Publishing Company, for their support and encouragement throughout the production of this book and for their unrelenting dedication to publishing meaningful resources for health care professionals.

I

Overview of Hospice

1

The Difference Between Hospice and Palliative Care

Hospice care has evolved over the past several decades and has always incorporated palliative care interventions. However, palliative care has taken on its own identity in American health care and is considered a specialty separate from hospice care. Although these two types of care are closely related, they are not the same. This chapter reviews the similarities and differences between hospice and palliative care.

After reading this chapter, you will be able to:

- Specify how hospice and palliative care differ
- Identify unique features of hospice care and palliative care
- Discuss hospice and palliative care as unique but interrelated specialty areas

HOSPICE CARE

Hospice care is widely recognized as a type of specialized care for terminally ill patients and their families that primarily takes place in the home (Coyle, 2015). By definition, hospice care is aimed at providing symptom management for patients with terminal illnesses and support for their families (Lanken et al., 2008). In hospice settings, the patient and family are considered to be the unit of care. Hospice care can be delivered in the patient's home, an inpatient hospice unit, a long-term care facility, or other settings. So, actually, the location of care is not what defines hospice care. Rather, according to Coyle (2015), hospice care incorporates the following:

- The care is specifically tailored to terminally ill patients.
- Hospice patients no longer receive curative treatments.
- Hospice patients can receive the Medicare hospice benefit.
- End-of-life concerns are addressed in a holistic manner.
- Patients receive skilled palliative care interventions.
- Care is provided mainly in the home.

Fast Facts in a Nutshell

Resources for the hospice and palliative nurse include:

- American Nurses Association
- End-of-Life Nursing Education Consortium
- Hospice and Palliative Credentialing Center
- Hospice and Palliative Nurses Association
- National Hospice and Palliative Care Organization
- The City of Hope

CHARACTERISTICS OF HOSPICE CARE

Hospice care is associated with terminality and there is often fear on the part of patients and families when the term is used. According to Hui et al. (2013), key concepts related to hospice include:

- Emphasis on symptom management
- Interprofessional care
- Caregiver involvement
- Bereavement services
- Six-month life expectancy
- Criteria-based determination of terminality/eligibility for hospice services
- Community-based care
- Availability of hospice inpatient services
- Availability of hospice volunteer and aide services

END-OF-LIFE PROTOCOLS

Hospice care, because it is specialized for end-of-life needs, involves certain specialized skills that pertain only to end-of-life situations. For example, several organizations have published position statements on end-of-life procedures such as withdrawal of mechanical ventilation (Lanken et al., 2008), the use of opioids at the end of life (Hospice and Palliative Nurses Association, 2004), and automatic implantable cardioverter-defibrillators (National Hospice and Palliative Care Organization, 2008). Protocols such as these underscore the unique skill-set of hospice nurses in ensuring comfort in the last moments of a patient's life. Several resources for end-of-life protocols and position statements include:

- The Hastings Center Guidelines (Berlinger, Jennings, & Wolf, 2013)
- National Hospice and Palliative Care Organization
- Hospice and Palliative Nurses Association
- American Nurses Association

BEREAVEMENT CARE

One feature of hospice care that sets it apart from palliative care is the incorporation of bereavement care for the family after the death of the patient. Bereavement care is a team effort and may involve phone calls or visits to the family members or caregivers for up to 1 year after the death of the patient. Many hospices also incorporate memorial services for bereavement families to help foster a sense of closure. Support groups are also regularly offered through hospices and may be specialized by the type of loss such as spousal loss or the loss of a child.

Fast Facts in a Nutshell

Palliative care has traditionally been outside of mainstream medicine but is gaining favor due to the growing prevalence of chronic illness (Coyle, 2015).

PALLIATIVE CARE

The World Health Organization (2016) defines palliative care as "an approach that improves the quality of life of patients and their families facing the problems associated with life-threatening illness, through the prevention and relief of suffering by means of early identification and impeccable assessment and treatment of pain and other problems, physical, psychosocial and spiritual."

Palliative care includes the management of symptoms such as pain, dyspnea, nausea and vomiting, fatigue, and others that interfere with the patient's ability to be comfortable. According to Coyle (2015), palliative care:

- Is a specialty
- Addresses spiritual, psychosocial, and cultural needs of patients and families
- Is available to patients in acute care, long-term care, or home settings
- Does not exclude curative treatments
- Is holistic
- Involves an interdisciplinary team
- Should be integrated into the plan of care for any serious, life-limiting condition at the time of diagnosis

Fast Facts in a Nutshell

Although "palliative care" is not specified as a Medicare benefit, Medicare Part B may cover some treatments and services that are considered palliative.

THE PALLIATIVE CARE NURSE

The expertise of the palliative care nurse is in the management of symptoms that disrupt the patient's and the family's quality of life. The palliative care nurse is an expert in using pharmacologic and nonpharmacologic measures to alleviate suffering within the context of either a curative plan of care or one that is strictly to promote comfort within the confines of the life-limiting disease. Coyle (2015) noted that the palliative care nurse strives to develop a close therapeutic relationship with the patient and family and serves as the liaison between the patient and the rest of the care team. The palliative care nurse may help broker the transition from "do everything" to "do everything to provide comfort and healing" (p. 6).

PROVISION OF PALLIATIVE CARE SERVICES

Unlike hospice services that are provided through an accredited hospice agency, palliative services may or may not be fully covered by Medicare or other health insurance plans. However, palliative care services are becoming more accepted and integrated into the continuum of care, and coverage options are changing rapidly.

Fast Facts in a Nutshell

For those interested in starting palliative care programs within organizations, the Center to Advance Palliative Care offers training, assistance, and tools. Find more information at www.capc.org.

Some hospitals have recognized the need for palliative services and have integrated this type of care. The Joint Commission began recognizing excellence in hospital-based palliative care in 2011. This type of certification recognizes that an organization (The Joint Commission, 2016):

- Has a formal palliative care program in place, led by an interdisciplinary team
- Has leadership that endorses and supports the palliative program
- Implements strategies to promote family engagement
- Offers coordinated care and services with an emphasis on interdisciplinary communication within the organization and with other agencies or providers involved in the patient's care
- Uses national, evidence-based guidelines to develop protocols for patient care

HOSPICE AND PALLIATIVE CARE SUMMARY

Table 1.1 contrasts key differences between hospice and palliative care.

Table 1.1

Differences Between Hospice and Palliative Care

Hospice Care	Palliative Care
A type of care for terminally ill and dying patients	A type of care aimed at promoting comfort for seriously ill patients whether their condition is terminal or not
Bereavement services are provided for up to 1 year after the death of the patient	Bereavement services are not always provided
Care is delivered primarily in the home	Care may be delivered in acute care, long-term care, or other settings
Patient chooses to forgo curative treatments	Palliative care is provided in conjunction with either curative or end-of-life treatments
Covered by the Hospice Medicare Benefit	May or may not be covered by Medicare or other health insurance plans
Life expectancy of patient is 6 months or less	Life expectancy is not a factor

CONCLUSION

In this chapter, the similarities and differences between hospice and palliative care were presented. The role of the nurse in each of these specialties was also reviewed. Although hospice care incorporates palliative care, palliative is a much broader type of care because it can be integrated into the plan of care for all seriously ill patients, and is not reserved for only those facing the end of life. For patients and families who are facing terminal illness, hospice care provides specialized services that are tailored to meet end-of-life needs, including bereavement support after the death of the patient.

References

Berlinger, N., Jennings, B., & Wolf, S. M. (2013). *The Hastings Center guidelines for decisions on life-sustaining treatment and care near the end of life: Revised and expanded second edition*. Oxford, UK: Oxford University Press.

Coyle, N. (2015). Introduction to palliative care. In B. R. Ferrell, N. Coyle, & J. A. Paice (Eds.), *Oxford Textbook of Palliative Nursing* (pp. 3–19). New York, NY: Oxford University Press.

Hospice and Palliative Nurses Association. (2004). HPNA position statement: Providing opioids at the end of life. Retrieved from http://www.hpna.org/filemaintenance_view.aspx?ID=27

Hui, D., De La Cruz, M., Mori, M., Parsons, H. A., Kwon, J. H., Torres-Vigil, I., . . . & Bruera, E. (2013). Concepts and definitions for "supportive care," "best supportive care," "palliative care," and "hospice care" in the published literature, dictionaries, and textbooks. *Supportive Care in Cancer, 21*(3), 659–685.

The Joint Commission. (2016). Facts about the Advanced Certification Program for Palliative Care. Retrieved from http://www.jointcommission.org/facts_about_palliative_care

Lanken, P. N., Terry, P. B., DeLisser, H. M., Fahy, B. F., Hansen-Flaschen, J., Heffner, J. E., . . . & Yankaskas, J. R. (2008). An official American Thoracic Society clinical policy statement: Palliative care for patients with respiratory diseases and critical illnesses. *American Journal of Respiratory and Critical Care Medicine, 177*(8), 912–927.

National Hospice and Palliative Care Organization. (2008). Understanding advanced directives. Retrieved from http://www.caringinfo.org/files/public/brochures/Understanding_Advance_Directives.pdf

World Health Organization. (2016). WHO definition of palliative care. Retrieved from http://www.who.int/cancer/palliative/definition/en

2

History and Evolution of Hospice in the United States

Today's hospice care is rooted in the end-of-life movement that came to the United States from Europe in the latter half of the 20th century. This chapter outlines the development of the modern hospice movement. It also discusses the related legislative changes that supported the growth of hospice in the United States.

After reading this chapter, you will be able to:

- Demonstrate an understanding of the origin of hospice care
- Identify turning points in the American hospice movement
- Discuss how research helped shape end-of-life practices
- Identify legislative changes that supported hospice care in the United States

HOSPICE IN THE UNITED STATES

Dame Cicely Saunders is credited as the foundress of the hospice movement. Saunders was trained as a nurse, social worker, and later as a physician. Her vision for hospice involved:

- Developing a humane and systematic approach to end-of-life care
- Devising an interdisciplinary approach to patient care

- Supporting the spiritual growth of patients and hospice staff
- Easing the pain and suffering involved in dying
  (Wright & Clark, 2012)

Saunders initially anticipated that hospice workers would be organized in a way that was similar to that of a religious order (Wright & Clark, 2012). But, as Saunders worked with others who were interested in improving end-of-life care, a more expansive hospice movement began to take shape. Saunders and her colleagues developed the document "Aim and Basis," which outlined the five premises of hospice care. With the scope of hospice defined, the first hospice, St. Christopher's, opened in London in 1967.

Fast Facts in a Nutshell

Saunders's passion for end-of-life care was partially fueled by her deep religious convictions and her belief that ministering to the dying was a religious calling (Wright & Clark, 2012).

Around the same time, the end-of-life movement was beginning to take shape in the United States. Dr. Elisabeth Kübler-Ross was a key researcher who advanced end-of-life conversations by:

- Conducting interviews with dying patients in the mid-1960s
- Identifying that certain themes emerged over and over
- Publishing her groundbreaking work *On Death & Dying* in 1969, which outlined the five stages that dying individuals go through when faced with a life-threatening condition. These were as follows:
  - Denial and Isolation
  - Anger
  - Bargaining
  - Depression
  - Acceptance

Slowly, health care professionals, researchers, and the public took interest in how death unfolded in America. Of special interest was how dying patients were treated in the hospital. In their book *Awareness of Dying*, Glaser and Strauss (1965) offered a telling account of how the technical expertise displayed by physicians and nurses contrasted with their interpersonal relations when working with dying patients. They found that health care professionals:

- Were quite uncomfortable working with dying patients
- Tended to avoid dying patients because they felt ill-prepared to discuss death
- Increased their own feelings of ineptitude and distress by avoiding and isolating dying patients

Fast Facts in a Nutshell

The Hospice Medicare Benefit covers services from doctors, nurses, nurse practitioners, nurses' aides, therapists, social workers, chaplains, and volunteers. Medical equipment, supplies, and medications that are related to the terminal illness are also covered. Respite care is available in an inpatient facility for up to 5 days each month (Centers for Medicare & Medicaid Services, 2015).

It was becoming clear to health professionals and the public that medical training was focused mainly on fighting disease and prolonging life. However, the growing interest in death and dying was already creating a shift in perspective and driving changes in health care. Throughout the 1970s and 1980s, hospice care initiatives grew rapidly. Thus, in:

- 1974: The Connecticut Hospice, Inc., the first hospice to open in the United States, began to provide end-of-life care (Simms, 2007)
- 1978: The National Cancer Institute provided funding to The Connecticut Hospice, Inc., "for the purposes of developing a national demonstration center for home care of the terminally ill and their families" (Committee on Finance, U.S. Senate, 1983, p. 2). By the end of 1978, there were 59 hospices in the United States (Greer, Mor, Sherwood, Morris, & Birnbaum, 1983)
- 1979: The Health Care Financing Administration funded an inquiry into the scope of hospice services, and the costs associated with this type of care (National Hospice and Palliative Care Organization, 2016; Simms, 2007)

- 1982: Congress approved a provision that covered hospice services under Medicare Part B. However, the provision included a sunset clause, which meant it would end in 1986 without congressional action
- 1983: The U.S. Senate report from the Committee on Finance, chaired by Senator Robert Dole, collected the data about hospice and ultimately reported that hospice care was more effective and cost-efficient than end-of-life care provided in the hospital setting. The average savings was $2,485 per patient, which in today's terms would be roughly $5,000 per patient
- 1984: The Joint Commission (formerly called the Joint Commission on Accreditation of Healthcare Organizations) began accrediting hospice organizations
- 1986: Recognizing the benefits of appropriate care for dying patients, Congress voted to make the Hospice Medicare Benefit permanent (National Hospice and Palliative Care Organization, 2015)
- 1991: Hospice care was recommended for inclusion in veterans' benefits (National Hospice and Palliative Care Organization, 2015)
- 1993: Hospice care became a nationally guaranteed benefit, and President Clinton recognized November as National Hospice Month (Clinton, 1993; National Hospice and Palliative Care Organization, 2015)
- 1994: The first certification examination for hospice nurses was administered through the Hospice and Palliative Credentialing Center (Hospice and Palliative Credentialing Center, 2014)
- 1997: The Balanced Budget Act included several provisions for hospice care, such as an updated payment structure, revised benefit periods, and expanded coverage for items and services related to the patient's terminal illness (Library of Congress, 2016)
- 2000: As a result of a collaborative effort between the City of Hope and the American Association of Colleges of Nursing, the End-of-Life Nursing Education Consortium (ELNEC) was launched with funding from the Robert Wood Johnson Foundation (ELNEC, 2012)
- 2001: The National Consensus Project, an interprofessional meeting to discuss end-of-life care in the United States, took place in New York City

- 2006: National Quality Forum (NQF) released "A national framework and preferred practices for palliative and hospice care quality: A consensus report"
- 2009: Updated clinical guidelines were created and released through a collaboration among the American Academy of Hospice and Palliative Medicine, the Center for the Advancement of Palliative Care, the Hospice and Palliative Nurses Association, and the National Hospice and Palliative Care Organization
- 2010: The Patient Protection and Affordable Care Act included provisions for the delivery of high-quality palliative and end-of-life care
- 2011: The Joint Commission launched "Advanced Palliative Care Certification" opportunities for qualifying health care organizations
- 2015: The Centers for Medicare & Medicaid Services introduced two new billing codes for advanced care planning provided for Medicare beneficiaries

Fast Facts in a Nutshell

The ELNEC curriculum was developed in 2000 to provide end-of-life training for registered nurses. Today, nearly 21,000 nurses and other health care professionals have attended ELNEC courses (American Association of Colleges of Nursing, 2015).

Numerous national and international efforts to improve care for terminally ill patients continue each year. Hospice care is available in every state in the United States and certification is available for registered nurses and advanced practice nurses. Hospice and palliative certification opportunities have also recently expanded into the areas of pediatric and perinatal nursing (Hospice and Palliative Credentialing Center, 2014).

Fast Facts in a Nutshell

The word "hospice" has the same linguistic root as the word "hospitality." In medieval times, a hospice was a place for travelers on a long journey to stay (National Hospice and Palliative Care Organization, 2015).

CONCLUSION

For the past 50 years, end-of-life care has been rapidly expanding in the United States, aided by the efforts of pioneers in the field and numerous legislative changes. The Hospice Medicare Benefit ensures access to hospice care for all Americans at the end of life. For nurses providing end-of-life care, certification is available and hospice care is now a recognized specialty.

References

American Association of Colleges of Nursing. (2015). ELNEC fact sheet. Retrieved from http://www.aacn.nche.edu/elnec/about/fact-sheet

Centers for Medicare & Medicaid Services. (2015). Medicare benefit policy manual. Retrieved from https://www.cms.gov/Regulations-and-Guidance/Guidance/Manuals/downloads/bp102c09.pdf

Clinton, W. J. (1993). Proclamation 6630: National hospice month, 1993 and 1994. Retrieved from http://www.presidency.ucsb.edu/ws/?pid=62503

Committee on Finance, U.S. Senate. (1983). Background materials on Medicare Hospice benefit. Retrieved from http://www.finance.senate.gov/imo/media/doc/sprt98-88.pdf

End-of-Life Nursing Education Consortium. (2012). History, statewide effort and recommendations for the future: Advancing palliative nursing care. Retrieved from http://www.aacn.nche.edu/elnec/publications/ELNEC-Monograph.pdf

Glaser, B. G., & Strauss, A. L. (1965). *Awareness of dying.* New Brunswick, NJ, Aldine Publishing.

Greer, D. S., Mor, V., Sherwood, S., Morris, J. N., & Birnbaum, H. (1983). National hospice study analysis plan. *Journal of Chronic Disease, 36*(11), 737–780.

Hospice and Palliative Credentialing Center. (2014). History of HPCC. Retrieved from http://hpcc.advancingexpertcare.org/about/history-of-hpcc

Kübler-Ross, E. (1969). *On death & dying: What the dying have to teach doctors, nurses, clergy, & their own families.* New York, NY: Scribner.

Library of Congress. (2016). H.R.2015—Balanced Budget Act of 1997. Retrieved from https://www.congress.gov/bill/105th-congress/house-bill/2015

National Hospice and Palliative Care Organization. (2015). History of hospice care. Retrieved from http://www.nhpco.org/history-hospice-care

National Hospice and Palliative Care Organization. (2016). Discharge from hospice services. Retrieved from http://www.nhpco.org/discharge-hospice-services

National Quality Forum. (2006). *A national framework and preferred practices for palliative and hospice care quality: A consensus report.* Retrieved from http://www.qualityforum.org/publications/2006/12/A_National

_Framework_and_Preferred_Practices_for_Palliative_and_Hospice_Care
_Quality.aspx

Simms, T. J. (2007). A perspective on the end of life: Hospice care. *Topics in Advanced Practice Nursing eJournal*. Retrieved from http://www.med scape.com/viewarticle/549702

Wright, M., & Clark, D. (2012). Cicely Saunders and the development of hospice palliative care. In H. Coward & K. I. Stajduhar (Eds.), *Religious understandings of a good death in hospice palliative care* (pp. 11–28). Albany: State University of New York Press.

3

Hospice Philosophy and the Role of the Nurse

The original Christian perspective that Sanders infused into hospice work ensured that each life was valued until its natural end and that each person received the highest quality of care until that time came (Wright & Clark, 2012). This outlook remains the bedrock for hospice nursing. However, over time, the development of scope and standards for hospice nursing has helped clarify and delineate the role of the hospice nurse.

After reading this chapter, you will be able to:

- Define the role of the nurse in hospice and palliative care
- Explain how patient care differs in the hospice setting
- Identify resources for hospice and palliative nurses

NURSING AND THE RELIEF OF HUMAN SUFFERING

The nurse has always been a central figure in the care of dying patients. But, over the past 40 years, the role of the hospice nurse in the United States has evolved considerably. Today, the hospice nurse is expected to have demonstrable expertise not only in the nursing care of patients who are actively dying, but also in palliative interventions.

Thus, the expertise of the hospice nurse is in alleviating symptoms, which aligns closely with the original goal of nursing as stated by

Florence Nightingale (1860) and has been reaffirmed by the American Nurses Association (ANA) in the following statement: "the aims of nursing actions (also nursing interventions) are to protect, promote, and optimize health; to prevent illness and injury; to alleviate suffering; and to advocate for individuals, families, communities, and populations" (2010a, p. 11).

HOSPICE NURSING AS A SPECIALTY AREA

In 1987, the first American organization for hospice nurses, the Hospice Nurses Association (HNA), was formed. This organization later created the National Board for Certification of Hospice Nurses (NBCHN) to develop a certification process for hospice nurses (Hospice and Palliative Nurses Association, 2004).

Fast Facts in a Nutshell

"The goal of hospice and palliative nursing is to promote and improve the patient's quality of life through the relief of suffering along the course of illness, through the death of the patient, and into the bereavement period for the family" (American Nurses Association/Hospice and Palliative Nurses Association, 2007, p. 1).

In 1994, the first certification exam for hospice nurses was offered. Those who passed this test earned the credential CRNH (Certified Registered Nurse Hospice; Hospice and Palliative Credentialing Center, 2014a).

In 1997, the HNA conducted a role delineation study and found that palliative care expertise was required of hospice nurses. Thus, in 1999, the NCBHN recognized this competency and offered the credential of CHPN (Certified Hospice and Palliative Nurse) to those who successfully completed the exam (Hospice and Palliative Nurses Association, 2004). The CRNH was retired in 2002, the same year that the credential CHPN was awarded accreditation by the American Board of Nursing Specialties (Hospice and Palliative Credentialing Center, 2014a). To more accurately represent the goals of these organizations, the HNA was renamed the Hospice and Palliative Nurses Association.

Question: Why should nurses become certified in hospice and palliative care?

Answer: Certification helps nurses:

- Demonstrate competency in pain and symptom management
- Improve end-of-life outcomes
- Validate nursing expertise
- Demonstrate a personal commitment to quality end-of-life care
(Hospice and Palliative Credentialing Center, 2014b)

The NCBHN also incorporated palliative care into its scope and was renamed the Hospice and Palliative Credentialing Center (HPCC). This board offers certification exams for administrators, licensed practical nurses, nursing assistants, registered nurses, and advanced practice nurses in hospice and palliative nursing. The hospice and palliative nursing examination for registered nurses covers seven areas that reflect required competencies:

1. Patient care: Life-limiting conditions in adult patients
2. Patient care: Pain management
3. Patient care: Symptom management
4. Care of the patient and family
5. Education and advocacy
6. Interdisciplinary/collaborative practice
7. Professional issues
   (Hospice and Palliative Credentialing Center, 2016)

The areas that are included on the HPCC certification exam align with the Scope and Standards for Hospice and Palliative Nursing, as outlined by the American Nurses Association/Hospice and Palliative Nurses Association (2007), which indicate that expertise in the following areas is required:

- Clinical judgment
- Advocacy and ethics
- Professionalism
- Collaboration
- Systems thinking
- Cultural competence

- Facilitation of learning
- Communication

STANDARDS OF PRACTICE

The American Nurses Association/Hospice and Palliative Nurses Association (2007) also outlined 16 standards of practice for hospice and palliative nursing. Six of these standards are related to professional practice:

Standard 1: Assessment
Standard 2: Diagnosis
Standard 3: Outcomes identification
Standard 4: Planning
Standard 5: Implementation
Standard 6: Evaluation

And 10 of the standards relate to professional performance:

Standard 7: Ethics
Standard 8: Education
Standard 9: Evidence-based practice and research
Standard 10: Quality of practice
Standard 11: Communication
Standard 12: Leadership
Standard 13: Collaboration
Standard 14: Professional practice evaluation
Standard 15: Resource utilization
Standard 16: Environmental health

Fast Facts in a Nutshell

In 2013, the ANA released a position statement on euthanasia, assisted suicide, and aid in dying. This and other position statements can be accessed at www.nursingworld.org/MainMenuCategories/EthicsStandards/Ethics-Position-Statements.

The ANA (2010b) released a position statement on the roles and responsibilities of the registered nurse in providing end-of-life care.

This document refers back to the ANA *Code of Ethics* (2001) and the Scope and Standards of Hospice and Palliative Nursing (American Nurses Association/Hospice and Palliative Nurses Association, 2007). Additionally, the position statement situates the End-of-Life Nursing Education Consortium (ELNEC) within the larger context of nursing education essentials. The ELNEC curriculum is offered worldwide and includes specialized content in nine areas pertinent to hospice and palliative nursing:

- Care at the end of life
- Pain management
- Symptom management
- Ethical and legal issues
- Cultural considerations
- Communication
- Grief, loss, and bereavement
- Achieving quality care at the end of life
- Preparation and care for the time of death

Question: Where can I find educational opportunities for end-of-life nursing?

Answer: The most widely recognized end-of-life training program for hospice and palliative nurses is ELNEC. More information can be found at www.aacn.nche.edu/elnec.

CONCLUSION

The role of the nurse in hospice and palliative care has expanded exponentially within the past 40 years. Today, certification for hospice and palliative nurses is available, and programs such as ELNEC provide a cohesive way of communicating the body of knowledge unique to this specialty. As a valued member of the hospice team, the nurse is responsible for coordinating the plan of care and must have the essential expertise to do so.

References

American Nurses Association. (2001). *Code of ethics for nurses with interpretive statements*. Silver Springs, MD: Nursesbooks.org.

American Nurses Association. (2010a). *Policy statement: The essence of the profession*. Silver Spring, MD: Nursesbooks.org.

American Nurses Association. (2010b). Position statement: Registered nurses' roles and responsibilities in providing expert care and counseling at the end of life. Retrieved from http://www.nursingworld.org/MainMenuCategories/EthicsStandards/Ethics-Position-Statements/etpain14426.pdf

American Nurses Association/Hospice and Palliative Nurses Association. (2007). *Hospice and palliative nursing: Scope and standards of practice*. Silver Spring, MD: Nursesbooks.org.

Hospice and Palliative Credentialing Center. (2014a). History of HPCC. Retrieved from http://hpcc.advancingexpertcare.org/about/history-of-hpcc

Hospice and Palliative Credentialing Center. (2014b). Why certification? Claiming and validating our expertise. Retrieved from http://hpcc.advancingexpertcare.org/competence/why-certification

Hospice and Palliative Credentialing Center. (2016). CHPN candidate handbook. Retrieved from http://www.goamp.com/Publications/candidateHandbooks/HPCC-CHPN-Handbook.pdf

Hospice and Palliative Nurses Association. (2004). *Statement on the scope and standards of hospice and palliative LPN/LVN practice*. Dubuque, IA: Kendall Hunt Publishing.

Nightingale, F. (1860). *What it is, and what it is not*. New York, NY: D. Appleton. Retrieved from http://digital.library.upenn.edu/women/nightingale/nursing/nursing.html

Wright, M., & Clark, D. (2012). Cicely Saunders and the development of hospice palliative care. In H. Coward & K. I. Stajduhar (Eds.), *Religious understandings of a good death in hospice palliative care* (pp. 11–28). Albany: State University of New York Press.

4

The Hospice Nurse as a Member of the Interdisciplinary Team

Hospice care is a holistic approach to the care of terminally ill patients and their families. Patients who are facing end-of-life issues have multidimensional needs and require the expertise of a team of professionals who work together to develop an individualized, comprehensive plan of care. This chapter reviews the roles of members of the hospice team and discusses the role of nurse as a team member.

After reading this chapter, you will be able to:

- Identify members of the interdisciplinary team and their functions
- Explain how the hospice team collaborates to develop a plan of care
- Discuss the role of the nurse within the interdisciplinary team

WHO'S ON THE TEAM?

First and foremost, the patient and family are the captains of the team. In every situation, the patient determines which care options are most in line with his or her end-of-life wishes. Within this context, the professionals on the hospice team, taking their lead from the patient and family, develop a plan of care that is specifically tailored to each patient. The Centers for Medicare & Medicaid Services (2015) outlined the services covered by members of the hospice team, including:

- **Nursing care:** These services "require the skills of a registered nurse (RN), or a licensed practical nurse (LPN) or a licensed vocational nurse (LVN), under the supervision of an RN, and must be reasonable and necessary for the palliation and management of the patient's terminal illness and related conditions" (p. 19).
- **Medical social services:** These services include assessment of the social and emotional factors related to the patient's terminal condition; assessment of the patient's medical and nursing needs, home situation, financial resources, and community resources; counseling services; and short-term social services for family members or caregivers with the goal of removing impediments to the provision of effective end-of-life care.
- **Physician services:** Within the interdisciplinary team, the hospice medical director must be prepared as either a doctor of osteopathic medicine (DO) or a medical doctor (MD). The hospice medical director must verify the patient's terminality and oversee medical care. The hospice medical director may complete the face-to-face visits intended to verify continued eligibility for hospice. The medical director may also serve as the attending physician for a hospice patient. The attending physician has "the most significant role in the determination and delivery of the individual's medical care" (p. 21). In some cases, a nurse practitioner may serve as the attending physician. The nurse practitioner must be employed by the hospice and the patient must have the option to receive care from a physician or a nurse practitioner. Nurse practitioners cannot certify or recertify terminality or prognosis.
- **Counseling services:** These services include the provision of emotional, psychosocial, and spiritual support for the patient and family. Bereavement counseling is also provided for the family for up to 1 year following the death of the patient.
- **Hospice aide and homemaker services:** Hospice aides provide personal care services as well as household services as needed to maintain a safe and clean environment for the patient. The hospice aide is assigned and supervised by the RN.

- **Physical therapy, occupational therapy, and speech therapy:** These services are "provided for purposes of symptom control or to enable the individual to maintain activities of daily living and basic functional skills" (p. 25).

Fast Facts in a Nutshell

The hospice interdisciplinary team addresses the biomedical, psychosocial, and spiritual care of the patient (Moore, Bastian, & Apenteng, 2015).

THE ROLE OF THE NURSE ON THE TEAM

Nursing education prepares nurses to work primarily in acute care settings and many hospices require a nurse to have at least 1 year of acute care experience prior to employment. Acute care experience is beneficial because, in hospice care, the nurse is alone in the patient's home and is expected to make decisions quickly and autonomously. However, working closely with all members of the interdisciplinary team on each case may be an adjustment for some nurses who have transitioned from the acute care environment.

Fast Facts in a Nutshell

Nurses who transition to working in hospice from an acute care setting bring transferrable skills but must develop expertise in palliative care (Rosser & King, 2003).

Within the interdisciplinary team, the hospice nurse is responsible for assessing the physical, emotional, and spiritual needs of patients and families, and for ensuring that the plan of care is carried out. Often, hospice nurses serve as the case manager (Moore et al., 2015) and are responsible for ensuring coordinated care delivery. As a case manager, the hospice nurse is responsible for:

- Providing reports on the patient's status and needs
- Coordinating care across disciplines

- Facilitating communication among team members, including the patient and family
- Ensuring quality care is provided throughout the hospice experience (Wittenberg-Lyles & Oliver, 2007)

Question: Where can I find information about hospice home care staffing?

Answer: The National Hospice and Palliative Care Organization (NHPCO, 2013) offers a free guide available at www.nhhpco.org/s -content/uploads/files/NHPCOStaffing_Guidelines.pdf.

In cases where the RN is not serving as case manager or is serving in the dual role of RN and case manager, some of the responsibilities of the hospice nurse include:

- Assessment of the patient's physical, spiritual, and psychosocial needs
- Assessment of the family's needs
- Implementation of the hospice care plan
- Administration of treatments
- Patient and family education
- Development of the nursing care plan
- Provision of high-quality, ethical nursing care
- Evaluation of effectiveness of palliative interventions
- Evaluation of nursing actions and other interventions
- Effective, professional communication with the patient, family, members of the interdisciplinary team, and community members

INTERDISCIPLINARY COMMUNICATION

The plan of care is typically established during interdisciplinary team meetings that occur as needed but no less frequently than every 15 days to develop a plan of care that meets the patient's physical, psychosocial, and spiritual needs (Centers for Medicare & Medicaid Services, 2008). During team meetings, members of the team communicate their understanding of the patient's condition and needs from their own disciplinary perspective. Effective communication facilitates quality patient care and underpins the team's ability to function cohesively (Doane, Stajduhar, Causton, Bidgood, & Cox, 2012).

The NHPCO (2010) has established a model for evaluating interdisciplinary team competency. The model helps hospice teams determine whether the team and individuals within the team are functioning at a novice, proficient, or expert level. (See Table 4.1.)

Fast Facts in a Nutshell

High-quality interdisciplinary team communication improves health outcomes for patients and families (Doane et al., 2012).

The NHPCO model can be used to develop a plan for moving a team from the "novice" to "expert" levels in each of the categories. Clearly, a well-functioning team is the bedrock of efficient and effective hospice care.

COORDINATING CARE WITHIN THE INTERDISCIPLINARY TEAM

Because hospice care is holistic and family centered, it is critical for the interdisciplinary team to function well. Although all members of the team are present at team meetings, discussion tends to focus largely on the biomedical aspects of care with nurses and doctors talking most frequently (Moore et al., 2015). To help ensure that all aspects of the patient's care are addressed and that the input of all members of the team is elicited, the nurse can:

- Encourage caregiver attendance and participation in team meetings
- Reduce role conflicts and interprofessional tensions through open communication strategies such as the use of one-across messages, which is a way of communicating without taking or relinquishing control of the conversation
- Ensure that everyone's contributions are taken seriously and that everyone is included in the decision-making process
- Be open to sharing negative patient experiences while ensuring that this results in unburdening for team members and allows for mutual support
  (Moore et al., 2015)

Table 4.1

Interdisciplinary Team Competency Grid

National Hospice and Palliative Care Organization

COMPETENCY	NOVICE	PROFICIENT	EXPERT
TEAM FUNCTION	■ Defines the interdisciplinary team	■ Collaborates with the interdisciplinary team to identify and meet patient/family identified needs	■ Models and teaches interdisciplinary team process and function to new team members
	■ Explains the difference between the medical model and the hospice philosophy of care	■ Assesses patient/family needs using patient/family-centered, holistic approach	■ Advocates for reframing the focus of care cooperatively with medical model practitioners/ organizations
	■ Describes the purpose and value of the interdisciplinary team to hospice care	■ Articulates the purpose and value of the interdisciplinary team to patients and families, fellow team members, and community	■ Serves as a role-model for interdisciplinary care, demonstrates expertise in utilizing the strengths of each discipline/ perspective and recognizing their limitations

■ Describes the purpose and value of the interdisciplinary team meeting	■ Participates in the interdisciplinary team meeting and considers the perspectives of all disciplines in the care planning process	■ Facilitates in-depth exploration of patient/family needs and engages in care planning processes that include all disciplines and address all patient/family identified needs
■ Identifies interdisciplinary team-related regulations and complies with them	■ Demonstrates compliance by putting regulations into context/practice	■ Keeps abreast of and educates colleagues about regulatory changes and assists in the development of organizational policy and process to ensure compliance
■ Describes ethical practice in end-of-life care	■ Participates in discussion of ethical issues and problem solving	■ Models ethical practice, is skilled in leading discussions about ethical issues and leads the problem-solving and resolution process
■ Identifies the elements of team process/team development (using B. Tuckman's [1965] "forming, storming, norming, performing" or other model of group development)	■ Describes the relevance of and applies group process/development to his/her interdisciplinary team	■ Observes group process and the development of his/her interdisciplinary team and reflects observations back to the group in efforts to further its development

(continued)

Table 4.1

Interdisciplinary Team Competency Grid (*continued*)

COMPETENCY	NOVICE	PROFICIENT	EXPERT
	■ Describes team discussion, team meeting, collaborative practice, evaluation, support, memorial and team activities	■ Participates in team discussion, team meeting, collaborative practice, support, memorial and team activities	■ Observes team discussion, meetings, collaborative practice, support, memorial and team activities; reflects observations back to the group and facilitates full integration of all members of the team
	■ Describes the process and rationale for interdisciplinary team evaluation	■ Participates in interdisciplinary team evaluation and identifies strategies to improve the team's work and collaboration	■ Synthesizes interdisciplinary team evaluation; notes trends; identifies need for improvement and progress toward improvement; facilitates improvements
WORKING WITH PATIENTS/FAMILIES	■ Articulates the role and contribution of each discipline to patient/family care	■ Promotes interdisciplinary care to meet identified patient/family needs	■ Helps patient/family (and colleagues) sort through complex and multi-dimensional needs to achieve identified goals

■ Describes the assessment process and methods of identifying patient/family-directed goals	■ Assesses and identifies desired patient/family-directed goals	■ Ensures that comprehensive and ongoing assessments are interdisciplinary and that they identify patient/family-directed goals
■ Describes the purpose of the plan of care in reflecting patient/family-centered goals and in directing the work of the interdisciplinary team	■ Participates in the development of the plan of care and uses it to guide interdisciplinary teamwork and practice	■ Helps team maintain focus on patient/family-identified goals in the plan of care (vs. their own); assists the interdisciplinary team (IDT) in revising the plan of care while maintaining patient/family-centered focus
■ Describes organizational protocols related to family closure	■ Provides appropriate closure with families in compliance with organizational protocols	■ Serves as a role model for fellow team members in providing closure that is firm yet sensitive to family needs
■ Describes patient/family-centered care, advocacy, and support	■ Promotes patient/family-centered care, advocacy, and support	■ Models interdisciplinary-focused patient/family-centered care, advocacy, and support
WORKING WITH TEAM MEMBERS ■ Identifies the specific role and responsibilities he/she has within the team	■ Identifies the strengths and limitations he/she brings to the team	■ Recognizes and utilizes professional and personal strengths, and values the diverse strengths of team members

(continued)

Table 4.1

Interdisciplinary Team Competency Grid (*continued*)

COMPETENCY	NOVICE	PROFICIENT	EXPERT
	■ Describes healthy and unhealthy boundaries	■ Maintains and promotes healthy boundaries	■ Confronts boundary issues within oneself and the team and challenges team to learn from experience
	■ Describes the importance of providing understanding and support to fellow team members	■ Demonstrates understanding and support in interactions with team members	■ Models behaviors of understanding and support and attends to the grief/loss needs of the team
COMMUNICATION	■ Keeps team members informed of patient/family needs/status	■ Utilizes collaborative team process to meet patient/family needs and effectively and efficiently applies them to care delivery	■ Clarifies thoughts and ideas; identifies and dispels misunderstandings around patient/family needs
	■ Describes the importance of being nonjudgmental in working with patients and families	■ Seeks, provides, and receives feedback without judgment	■ Confronts judgment within oneself and the team and challenges team to learn from experience

QUALITIES OF A
HIGH-FUNCTIONING
TEAM MEMBER

- Reports relevant patient/family information in a professional, efficient manner

- Collaborates with fellow team members to schedule visits with patient/family and reports outcomes of visits to other team members

- Identifies urgent and/or changing needs and communicates them to the team

- Documents key patient/family information in a timely, accurate, compliant manner that addresses needs identified in the plan of care

- Summarizes relevant patient/family information in a professional, efficient manner, ensuring the inclusion of all team members and volunteers

- Coordinates visits with team members to best meet patient/family-identified needs

- Collaborates with team members to determine a timely and effective response to urgent/changing needs

- Summarizes key patient/family information in a manner that reflects care and collaboration with team members to implement and continually revise the plan of care

- Provides analysis of relevant patient/family information in a professional, efficient manner for team members and volunteers

- Engages team in evaluation of its productivity, efficiency, and effectiveness in implementing the plan of care

- Leads team in developing timely and effective response to urgent/changing needs and ensures plan of care is being followed

- Provides guidance to fellow team members about the documentation process and its relevance to their work and serves as a key organizational resource to evaluate and guide the development of systems and processes to facilitate efficient documentation

(continued)

Table 4.1

Interdisciplinary Team Competency Grid *(continued)*

COMPETENCY	NOVICE	PROFICIENT	EXPERT
	■ Describes the behaviors of punctuality, follow through, and accountability with respect to team collaboration	■ Is punctual, follows through, and is accountable to other team members	■ Models appropriate time management, shares strategies, and coaches peers
	■ Describes the importance and value of courtesy, respect, inclusiveness, and nonjudgment with respect to patients/families and fellow team members	■ Demonstrates courtesy, respect, inclusiveness, and nonjudgment with respect to patients/families and fellow team members	■ Works collaboratively with team members to expand understanding of inclusion and leads the development of new strategies/approaches as indicated
	■ Participates in professional development opportunities in professional discipline and interdisciplinary team development	■ Assists in identifying, creating, and/or teaching professional development and interdisciplinary team development activities	■ Leads, teaches, and assists in the evaluation of professional development and interdisciplinary team development activities
	■ Identifies and describes own practice approaches	■ Actively develops and enhances own practice approaches through supervision, mentoring, coaching, or related activities	■ Develops self-reflective ability to monitor own practice approach(es) and models self-reflection to team members

COLLABORATIVE PROBLEM SOLVING		
• Describes best practices in own discipline and interdisciplinary team practice	• Applies best practices in own discipline to care delivery and interdisciplinary team practice	• Leads the identification and creation of care delivery processes to further the development of the interdisciplinary team
• Describes critical thinking	• Utilizes critical thinking	• Assesses the effectiveness of critical thinking to the team process and patient/family outcomes
• Describes situations that lead to, and identifies ways people respond to, conflict	• Articulates the value/role of team conflict and views it as opportunity to enhance team function	• Models and coaches team in effective conflict resolution
• Identifies problems in team function and practice	• Participates in problem solving about team function and process	• Models problem-solving skills in addressing problems in team function and process
• Identifies common pitfalls to teamwork (e.g., discipline-ism, lone ranger-ism, martyr-ism*)	• Practices teamwork without yielding to pitfalls	• Addresses pitfalls to team work (i.e., discipline-ism, lone ranger-ism, martyr-ism*) when observed/experienced

* DEFINITIONS:

Discipline-ism

• Identification with one's own specialty in a way that presumes one's own discipline has more value than the others or that diminishes the contributions of other disciplines

• Lack of collaboration or failure to recognize the value of perspectives from other disciplines and a team approach

(continued)

Table 4.1

Interdisciplinary Team Competency Grid (continued)

- Domination or control due to the influence or approach of members in particular disciplines
- Limiting opportunities for input from other disciplines
- Failure to convey value of other disciplines to patients and families

Lone-Ranger-ism

- Acting independently, without collaboration or input from the interdisciplinary team
- Behavior that results in isolation or lack of fellowship, responsibility, and accountability of all team members toward each other
- Demonstrates lack of ability to participate as a team member/work with team; possibly a result of discomfort sharing attention or success with others
- Acting and believing that "I can do it alone"

Martyr-ism

- Acting and believing that "I have to carry the burden because no one else can do what I do," resulting in perceived sacrifice of self
- Behavior indicates need for attention, need for recognition, or inability to practice within appropriate professional boundaries
- Behavior reflects an exaggerated sense of self-importance and skill
- Inability (or lack of willingness) to identify and utilize appropriate resources

Functional Utilization of the Interdisciplinary Team Competency

NHPCO'S Competency Subcommittee (of its Professional Education Committee) has identified the following functional uses for the *Interdisciplinary Team Competency:*

- Employee Selection/Hiring: Develop job-specific criteria for IDT-related positions in your organization utilizing the competency and design interview questions to assess candidate's skills.
- Orientation Programs: Utilize the "novice" indicators in planning your orientation program and to ensure that incoming staff understand the interdisciplinary team model.
- Ongoing Education: Utilize the competencies to develop an annual education plan, developing seminars and workshops to teach IDT members new skills.
- Professional Development: Use the novice, proficient, and expert levels to develop an individual's professional development plan or to create a "career ladder" for IDT members.
- Performance Appraisals: Incorporate relevant IDT competency indicators into annual performance appraisal processes, using them to measure an individual's performance of specific job skills.

National Hospice & Palliative Care Organization (2010). Used with permission.

CONCLUSION

Within the interdisciplinary team, the nurse coordinates the plan of care and helps facilitate effective communication to foster quality end-of-life care. Key competencies for the well-functioning interdisciplinary team include effective communication and collaboration.

References

Centers for Medicare & Medicaid Services. (2008). Medicare & Medicaid programs: Hospice conditions of participation. Retrieved from https://www.gpo.gov/fdsys/pkg/FR-2008-06-05/pdf/08-1305.pdf

Centers for Medicare & Medicaid Services. (2015). Local Coverage Determination (LCD): Hospice—Determining terminal status (L33393). Retrieved from https://www.cms.gov/medicare-coverage-database/details/lcd-details.aspx?LCDId=33393&ver=2&kc=59c12399-6&bc=AAAAAAQAAAAAAA%3d%3d&#0

Doane, G. H., Stajduhar, K., Causton, E., Bidgood, D., & Cox, A. (2012). End-of-life care and interprofessional communication: Not simply a matter of "more." *Health & Interprofessional Practice*, *1*(3), 1–14. doi:10.7772/2159-1253.1028

Moore, A. R., Bastian, R. G., & Apenteng, B. A. (2015). Communication within hospice interdisciplinary teams: A narrative review. *American Journal of Hospice & Palliative Medicine*. Advance online publication. doi:10.1177/1049909115613315

National Hospice and Palliative Care Organization. (2010). Interdisciplinary competency grid. Retrieved from http://www.nhpco.org/sites/default/files/public/education/Competency_level_grid_final.pdf

National Hospice and Palliative Care Organization. (2013). Staffing guidelines for hospice care teams. Retrieved from http://www.nhhpco.org/s-content/uploads/files/NHPCOStaffing_Guidelines.pdf

Rosser, M., & King, L. (2003). Transition experiences of qualified nurses moving into hospice nursing. *Journal of Advanced Nursing*, *43*(2), 206–215. Retrieved from http://onlinelibrary.wiley.com/journal/10.1111/(ISSN)1365-2648

Tuckman, B. W. (1965). Developmental sequence in small groups. *Psychological Bulletin*, *63*(6), 384.

Wittenberg-Lyles, E. M., & Oliver, D. P. (2007). The power of interdisciplinary collaboration in hospice. *Progress in Palliative Care*, *15*(1), 6–12.

II

The Nuts and Bolts of Hospice Nursing

5

Establishing Goals of Care

Hospice nurses are experts at supporting patients and their families during the transition from curative care to end-of-life care. They partner with families to ensure their loved ones' wishes are honored and periodically reestablish goals of care if the patient's condition improves or declines. This chapter addresses the role of the hospice nurse in establishing goals of care and facilitating difficult conversations with patients and families.

After reading this chapter, you will be able to:

- Establish goals of care with patients and families
- Manage difficult conversations regarding end-of-life care
- Help facilitate family conversations regarding the patient's end-of-life wishes and resolve family conflicts regarding end-of-life care

ESTABLISHING AND REESTABLISHING GOALS OF CARE

Prior to a referral to hospice, many patients have lived with chronic illness and disability for some time. Patients and their families may have had conversations with the primary care provider regarding goals of care and recommended treatments. Referral for hospice services is an indication that health care providers and patients feel that the goals of care have shifted primarily to symptom management, rather than curative care.

Knowing that previously stated end-of-life wishes sometimes change as patients actually face a terminal disease, hospice nurses support patients as they establish or reestablish goals within the context of the disease process. For example, a patient whose living will previously included mechanical ventilation may decide that such intervention is no longer congruent with his or her end-of-life wishes. Focused conversations open the door to determining whether patients' goals are consistent with hospice philosophy.

Establishing goals of care is a learned skill that requires excellent communication skills and empathy for the patient's circumstances. Conversations regarding goals of care can often begin by asking the patient whether he or she has a living will or an advance directive. Patients and families are sometimes unclear on the differences between these terms, so hospice nurses can clarify them using definitions provided by the National Hospice and Palliative Care Organization (2008). (See Figure 5.1.)

If a patient has a living will or has established medical power of attorney, this is an indication that the patient has considered what type of end-of-life care he or she might want. Importantly, living wills are created by patients when they are well and attempting to envision what type of care they might want in the event of a medical emergency.

One way that a patient may document end-of-life wishes is by using Physician Orders for Life-Sustaining Treatment (POLST), which:

- Document a plan of care that is created through a serious conversation between a health care provider and patient
- Are intended for patients who have a life-limiting disease and a life expectancy of less than 1 year (Bomba, Kemp, & Black, 2012)
- Follow patients throughout all care settings, such as home care, in-hospital care, and long-term care facilities
- Are typically printed on brightly colored paper so that they stand out in a chart (for a POLST example, see the Appendix)

Question: Where can I find more information about POLST?
Answer: Visit the National POLST website at www.polst.org/about-the-national-polst-paradigm/what-is-polst.

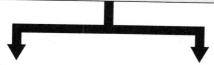

Advance Directives (ADs)

Legal documents that patients design to make their end-of-life (EOL) wishes known in the event that they are not able to communicate on their own. ADs include living wills and medical power of attorney (POA) documents.

Living Wills

A written statement created by a patient when he or she is well that communicates the type of care he or she would want if unable to communicate due to illness. This type of AD becomes effective only if the patient is unable to express his or her own wishes.

Medical Power of Attorney

In this type of AD, a patient designates another person to make medication decisions for him or her if he or she is unable to make his or her own decisions due to illness. Other terms used interchangeably include "health care proxy," "surrogate," or "health care agent."

Figure 5.1 Advance directives.

For patients who have already had conversations about their wishes with their families and health care providers, reaffirming goals helps to establish a therapeutic relationship with the patient and ensure that the plan of care is consistent with the patient's wishes. For patients who have not discussed their end-of-life wishes with their families or health care providers, the conversation can be more challenging and may involve reviewing or breaking bad news to the patient and the family. Several models for approaching difficult patient conversations have been published.

MANAGING DIFFICULT CONVERSATIONS

Hospice nurses working with terminally ill patients share bad news with patients and families on a regular basis. Although the patient may be aware of the terminal diagnosis and may have opted to forgo life-sustaining treatment, the illness trajectory may still catch patients off guard. One model of sharing serious news is the SPIKES model (Baile et al., 2000) that comprises the following six steps:

S—Setting: The setting should be private and anyone whom the patient wants to have there should be present. The professional should sit down, take the conversation slowly, and establish a therapeutic rapport with the patient and family. The provider should also limit interruptions by asking those present to turn off cell phones and pagers.

P–Perceptions: The professional should establish what the patient and family already know about the medical condition and their expectations, hopes, and fears.

I—Invitation: The professional should establish what the patient and family want to know and elicit an invitation to share more information.

K—Knowledge sharing: The professional should share the information with the patient and family after explaining that the news is serious. Medical jargon should be avoided and the professional should stop talking periodically to check the patient's understanding.

E—Emotions: After sharing the serious news, the professional should assess the patient and family's emotional state and identify their emotions (e.g., sadness, shock, or anger). The professional should then try to connect the emotion to the circumstances, and express that to the patient and family as a way of expressing empathy and validating how difficult it is to receive unwanted news.

S–Strategy and Summary: The professional should proceed to discussing interventions only if the patient and family are ready to consider them. The patient and family may feel uncertain about what to do or may seek guidance from the professional. Here, the professional can provide direction if indicated but should always engage in shared decision making with patients and families to ensure that their goals are honored.

Fast Facts in a Nutshell

An excellent resource for facilitating family discussion about the patient's end-of-life wishes is available from *The Conversation Project*. More information about the project and a family starter kit can be found at www.theconversationproject.org.

For patients who had not previously considered their end-of-life wishes but are faced with the news of declining health, the hospice nurse should work with the hospice social worker to facilitate a conversation between the patient and family members regarding end-of-life care. This conversation should center on the following:

- What does the patient value as he or she faces terminal illness?
- How should decisions regarding care be made?
- Where and how would the patient prefer to spend his or her last days?

FACILITATING FAMILY CONVERSATIONS

When patients choose hospice care, a decision is made to forgo curative treatment and focus care efforts on comfort. Hospice nurses are experts at devising plans of care that meet the patient's stated needs. However, sometimes family members do not agree with the patient's wishes or there is conflict among family members about what is the best course of action. In these situations, the hospice nurse partners with members of the interdisciplinary team to establish common goals and resolve conflict when necessary.

When working with family, the hospice nurse:

- Takes a family-centered approach, recognizing the expertise of the family in regard to care of the patient
- Works collaboratively with the family; no hierarchy can exist because the patient and the family are considered the unit of care (Wittenberg-Lyles, Goldsmith, Ferrell, & Ragan, 2013)
- Carefully observes family communication patterns, family structure, and the emergence of conflicts

Fast Facts in a Nutshell

"Patient- and family-centered care is an approach to the planning, delivery, and evaluation of health care that is grounded in mutually beneficial partnerships among health care providers, patients, and families" (Institute for Patient- and Family-Centered Care, 2010, para. 1).

Conflict can arise within a family when a loved one is dying because serious illness and death are significant stressors on a family's well-being and established routines. When faced with crisis, family adaptation can be facilitated by the hospice team. First, the source or sources of the conflict must be identified. According to the NSW Department of Health (2010), numerous factors can contribute to end-of-life conflict, including:

- Conflict between the patient and the health care provider
- Conflict within the health care team
- Emotional responses to dying and loss
- Difficulty with conveying poor prognosis and predicting death
- Inadequate advanced care planning
- Impact of external factors such as inadequacy of rooms to hold family conferences, gaps in documentation of end-of-life discussions, and geographic distance of family members
- Cross-cultural issues such as extended families, use of interpreters, demands to continue aggressive care due to cultural or religious beliefs, gender-based roles, and misinterpreting verbal and nonverbal communication
- Risk management, which involves fear of legal repercussions related to engaging in conversations about futile care

Fast Facts in a Nutshell

In a study by Prouty, Fischer, Purdom, Cobos, and Helmeke (2016), spiritual coping led to increased family communication and improved family functioning.

FAMILY STRESS AND RESILIENCE

Families, based on their histories of cohesiveness or lack of cohesiveness, have a certain capacity to weather crises. When facing a stressor such as the loss of a loved one, families engage in the active processes of adapting to the loss within the limits of their own capacity to do so (Patterson, 2002). Based on several well-established theories of family stress and resilience, Patterson (2002) noted that:

- Community and culture contribute to a family's ability to cope with stress
- The process of adapting to a stressor may require a restructuring of the family's beliefs and values

- Many families engage in stable coping patterns, but some families do not have the capacity for adjustment
- Family crisis may result when families do not have the ability to adjust to stressors
- When facing crises, families may develop resilience and successfully manage challenges or family processes may be further disrupted, leading to poor outcomes

Hospice nurses are keenly aware that what affects one member of the family affects the entire family system. The hospice nurse works closely with the hospice social worker and hospice chaplain to assess the family's risk for crisis. Family meetings may be an effective way for the hospice team to support families through conflict and crisis.

FAMILY MEETINGS

The goal of a family meeting is to facilitate collaboration and communication between the family and the health care team. Along with other members of the hospice team, during a family meeting, the hospice nurse:

- Supports the family's understanding of the patient's current condition
- Helps relieve the family's uncertainty regarding the prognosis
- Helps translate medical terminology and jargon
- Supports and reassures family members
- Helps mediate family conflict
  (Wittenberg-Lyles et al., 2013)

CONCLUSION

In this chapter, the role of the hospice nurse in establishing and reaffirming a patient's end-of-life wishes was discussed. Additionally, the nurse's role in communicating changes in the patient's condition was reviewed. The chapter ended with a discussion of how to identify and intervene appropriately, along with other members of the hospice team, during times of family conflict. This information provides a strong foundation for hospice nurses establishing goals of care with patients and families and ensuring agreement regarding the plan of care.

References

Baile, W. F., Buckman, R., Lenzl, R., Global, G., Beale, E. A., & Kudelka, A. P. (2000). SPIKES: A six-step protocol for delivering bad news: Application to the patient with cancer. *The Oncologist, 5*(4), 302–311. doi:10.1634/theon cologist.5-4-302

Bomba, P., Kemp, M., & Black, J. S. (2012). POLST: An improvement over traditional advance directives. *Cleveland Clinic Journal of Medicine, 79*(7), 457–464. doi:10.3949/ccjm.79a.11098

Institute for Patient- and Family-Centered Care. (2010). What is patient- and family-centered health care? Retrieved from http://www.ipfcc.org/about/pfcc.html

National Hospice and Palliative Care Organization. (2008). Understanding advance directives. Retrieved from http://www.caringinfo.org/files/public/brochures/Understanding_Advance_Directives.pdf

NSW Department of Health. (2010). Conflict resolution in end-of-life settings (CRELS). Retrieved from http://www.health.nsw.gov.au/patients/acp/Publications/conflict-resolution.pdf

Patterson, J. M. (2002). Integrating family resilience and family stress theory. *Journal of Marriage and Family, 64*(2), 349–360. Retrieved from http://onlinelibrary.wiley.com/journal/10.1111/(ISSN)1741-3737

Prouty, A. M., Fischer, J., Purdom, A., Cobos, E., & Helmeke, K. B. (2016). Spiritual coping: A gateway to enhancing family communication during cancer treatment. *Journal of Religion and Health, 55*(1), 269–287. doi:10.1007/s10943-015-0108-4

Wittenberg-Lyles, E., Goldsmith, J., Ferrell, B., & Ragan, S. (2013). *Communication in palliative nursing.* New York, NY: Oxford University Press.

6

Establishing Hospice Eligibility

At the time of admission, and on an ongoing basis, the hospice nurse is responsible for assessing the patient's condition and documenting that the patient continues to meet established criteria for hospice care. This chapter discusses several guidelines and prognostic tools.

After reading this chapter, you will be able to:

- Identify hospice eligibility guidelines
- Discuss tools used to support the need for end-of-life care
- Determine eligibility for hospice services

Question: What if my patient is not Medicare-eligible?
Answer: The hospice social worker will work closely with individuals who have private insurance or no insurance to establish how care will be covered and to connect patients and their families with needed resources.

GUIDELINES AND ASSESSMENT TOOLS

Most commonly, patients utilize the Hospice Medicare Benefit to cover hospice services. According to the Centers for Medicare & Medicaid

Services (2015b), to receive this benefit, patients must be eligible for Medicare Part A and:

- Accept hospice care instead of curative treatments
- Sign a statement choosing hospice care and revoking Medicare benefits for curative treatment of the terminal condition
- Receive certification of terminality (life expectancy of 6 months or less) from *both* the primary care physician *and* the hospice medical director

Question: Where can my patients find reliable information about the Hospice Medicare Benefit?
Answer: Patients and their families can go to Medicare.gov and search for "hospice" in the search bar.

Other criteria are also used to support terminality and eligibility for services and should be documented in the patient's record. For example, Local Coverage Determination (LCD) is used by the National Government Services to determine eligibility for hospice care (Jones, Harrington, & Mueller, 2013). These guidelines (Centers for Medicare & Medicaid Services, 2015a) specify criteria for:

- Decline in clinical status
- Nondisease-specific baseline guidelines
- Disease-specific guidelines

A summary of Medicare's LCD for hospice service eligibility is shown in Table 6.1.

The LCD guidelines reference several other tools that are used to determine terminality. Some of these tools include:

- **The Functional Assessment Staging Test (FAST©) Scale:** This scale was developed as an evaluation tool for patients who have dementia (Reisberg, 1987). Health care professionals use the FAST Scale to document a patient's functional status according to the seven stages included in the scale. A score of 1 indicates no impairment; 2 to 5 indicates mild to moderate impairment; 6 to 7 indicates moderately severe to severe impairment

Table 6.1

Medicare's Local Coverage Determination for Hospice Eligibility

Key points regarding recertification	■ Document decline as needed but not less than every 15 days ■ Recertification is based on ongoing documented evidence of decline and patient instability. If the patient's condition partially meets or does not meet LCD criteria, consider physician assessment, diagnosis change, and/or discharge.
Types of disease trajectory	■ Rapid decline: short period of steady decline (e.g., cancer) ■ Saw-toothed decline: episodes of exacerbations, never back to previous baseline (e.g., COPD) ■ Slow insidious decline: prolonged dwindling (e.g., dementia, frailty)
Key questions to ponder	Pain and symptom management ■ What are the symptoms we are managing? What does it take to keep them under control? ■ How often are these symptoms escalating or the patient is having a crisis? Disease progression/change in quality of life ■ What evidence of decline are we seeing, reading, observing (e.g., food intake, weight, physical assessment, arm circumference, mental status, change in medications/O_2)? ■ What is the patient/family telling us about decline (e.g., stamina, ADL, sleep/rest, social engagement, activities, symptoms, pain, psychospiritual issues)? LCD criteria ■ Does the patient still meet LCD guidelines? ■ Does the disease trajectory (pattern and momentum of decline) still reflect a terminal condition? Instability ■ Is the patient relatively stable? What would happen if hospice services were removed? ■ Will the improvement be sustained? What is the course of care and caregiver challenge?

(continued)

Table 6.1

Medicare's Local Coverage Determination for Hospice Eligibility (*continued*)

Clinical status guidelines (use if there are no LCD-specific disease guidelines)	■ Intractable serious infections: pneumonia, pyelonephritis, septicemia, recurrent fevers ■ Progressive inanition (exhaustion, lethargy) evidenced by: ■ >10% ↓ Weight in past 6 mo or body mass index G22 kg/m² (not due to depression/diuretics) ■ ↓ Mid-arm circumference (acromion [shoulder] to olecranon [elbow]) or abdominal girth ■ ↓ Skin turgor, ill-fitting clothes, increasing skin folds if weight not documented ■ Laboratory: albumin G2.5, cholesterol ■ Dysphagia with measured aspiration (e.g., history of choking/gagging with feeding) or intake as evidence by decreasing cups of food consumed ■ Symptoms (intractable/poorly responsive): dyspnea with ↑ respiratory rate; cough; nausea/vomiting; diarrhea; pain requiring ↑ doses of major analgesics ■ Signs: systolic blood pressure >90 mm Hg or ↑ postural hypotension; ascites; edema; venous, arterial, lymphatic obstruction; weakness; ↓ level of consciousness ■ Laboratory: ↑ P_{CO_2} or ↓ PO_2/Sao_2; ↑ calcium, creatinine or liver function; ↑↓↑ serum Na^+ or K^+ ■ ↓ PPS due to disease progression ■ ↓ FAST: 7a 96 words; 7b ~1 word; unable to: walk-7c, sit up-7d, smile-7e, hold head up-7f ■ ↓ ADL: ambulation, bathing, continence, dressing, feeding, transfer ■ Progressive stage 3–4 pressure ulcers despite optimal care ■ ↑ ED visits, hospitalization, physician visits related to 1st diagnosis prior to election of hospice
Baseline to use with specific disease guidelines	■ Documented clinical progression of disease: multiple ED visits, hospitalizations, home visits ■ PPS < 70% (PPS for stroke or HIV < 50%) ■ Partial/full dependence for 2+ ADLs: ambulation, bathing, continence, dressing, feeding, transfer ■ Significant comorbidities, eg, congestive heart failure, COPD, DM, ischemic heart, renal, liver, HIV, dementia, neurological (cerebrovascular accident, amyotrophic lateral sclerosis, Parkinson disease), autoimmune (lupus, rheumatoid arthritis)

(*continued*)

Table 6.1

Medicare's Local Coverage Determination for Hospice Eligibility (*continued*)

- Receiving supportive, palliative, comfort care or treatment to comfort/improve functional level (e.g., intravenous fluids, nasogastric tubes, transfusions, palliative chemotherapy, or radiation therapy)

ADL, activities of daily living; COPD, chronic obstructive pulmonary disease; DM, diabetes mellitus; ED, emergency department; LCD, Local Coverage Determination; P_{CO_2}, partial pressure of carbon dioxide; PO_2, partial pressure of oxygen; PPS, Palliative Performance Scale; Sao$_2$, arterial oxygen saturation.

(Reisberg et al., 1996). FAST Scale scores of 6 to 7 have been associated with increased mortality (Sampson, Leurent, Blanchard, Jones, & King, 2013). Patients who have dementia must be at Stage 7 to be eligible for hospice services. (The FAST Scale is included in the Appendix.)

- **The Karnofsky Scale:** This scale was first developed in the 1940s as a way to measure a patient's status throughout cancer treatment (Karnofsky & Burchenal, 1949; Timmerman, 2012). It has been extensively tested and is a reliable and valid measure of performance status. This scale is also useful for prognostication purposes (Abernethy, Shelby-James, Fazekas, Woods, & Currow, 2005); a low score is associated with a poor prognosis. However, the scale indicates that a patient with a score of less than or equal to 30 requires hospitalization (see Appendix for Karnofsky Scale). Most hospice and palliative clinicians do not use the scale to determine the need for hospitalization, but rather, to assess and document declining health status. Another tool, the Palliative Performance Scale (PPS), is a modified version of the Karnofsky Performance Scale and is widely used in hospice and palliative settings.

- **The Palliative Performance Scale© (PPS):** This scale is based on the Karnofsky Performance Scale and is meant to be used to develop a clinical snapshot of the patient's status at a given time. Reassessment of the patient's condition over time allows clinicians to monitor changes in the patient's status using a standardized tool that helps establish prognosis. As scores decrease from 100% (no evidence of disease) to 0% (death), the patient's mortality risk increases (Anderson, Downing, Hill, Casorso, & Lerch, 1996).

The PPS has been modified (Victoria Hospice Society, 2001), and the second version is a useful clinical tool for prognostication (Chan, Wu, & Chan, 2013). For nonspecific terminal illness, a PPS score of less than or equal to 70% supports hospice admission. For patients who have a diagnosis of cerebrovascular accident (CVA) or HIV, a score of less than or equal to 50% supports hospice admission (Jones et al., 2013). (The PPSv2 [PPS version 2] is included in the Appendix.)

- **The Eastern Cooperative Oncology Group (ECOG) Performance Scale:** This scale is used to determine the progression of a patient's disease on a scale from 0 (no restriction) to 5 (dead). Although an ECOG score is not specifically required for hospice admission, a score of more than or equal to 2 is predictive of a prognosis of 6 months or less (Wright & Kinzbrunner, 2011).

Fast Facts in a Nutshell

Medicare services for conditions unrelated to the terminal condition are still available to patients who choose hospice. Also, patients who agree to hospice services but then choose to pursue curative treatment for the terminal illness may revoke the hospice benefit in order to do so (Centers for Medicare & Medicare Services, 2015a).

CONCLUSION

In this chapter, eligibility criteria for hospice services were reviewed. Specifically, requirements for meeting the criteria to access the Medicare Hospice Benefit were discussed. Also, numerous tools for supporting terminality were reviewed individually. Use of these tools will help hospice nurses document how patients meet Medicare's LCD guidelines for hospice service on admission and on an ongoing basis.

References

Abernethy, A. P., Shelby-James, T., Fazekas, B. S., Woods, D., & Currow, D. C. (2005). The Australia-modified Karnofsky Performance Status (AKPS) scale: A revised scale for contemporary palliative care clinical practice. *BMC Palliative Care, 4*(7). doi:10.1186/1472-684X-4-7

Anderson, F., Downing, M., Hill, J., Casorso, L., & Lerch, N. (1996). Palliative Performance Scale (PPS): A new tool. *Journal of Palliative Care*, *12*(1), 5–11.

Centers for Medicare & Medicaid Services. (2015a). Medicare benefit policy manual. Retrieved from https://www.cms.gov/Regulations-and-Guidance/Guidance/Manuals/downloads/bp102c09.pdf

Centers for Medicare & Medicaid Services. (2015b). Local Coverage Determination (LCD): Hospice—Determining terminal status (L33393). Retrieved from https://www.cms.gov/medicare-coverage-database/details/lcd-details.aspx?LCDId=33393&ver=2&kc=59c12399-6&bc=AAAAAAQAAAAAAA%3d%3d&#0

Chan, E. Y., Wu, H. Y., & Chan, Y. H. (2013). Revisiting the Palliative Performance Scale: Change in scores during disease trajectory predicts survival. *Palliative Medicine*, *27*(4), 367–374. doi:10.1177/0269216312451613

Jones, M., Harrington, T., & Mueller, G. (2013). Hospice admission eligibility: A staff education project. *Journal of Hospice & Palliative Nursing*, *15*(2), 114–122. doi:10.1097/NJH.0b013e31826d743c

Karnofsky, D. A., & Burchenal, J. H. (1949). The clinical evaluation of chemotherapeutic agents in cancer. In C. M. MacLeod (Ed.), *Evaluation of chemotherapeutic agents*. New York, NY: Columbia University Press.

Reisberg, B. (1987). Functional assessment staging (FAST). *Psychopharmacology Bulletin*, *24*(4), 653–659. Retrieved from https://www.researchgate.net/journal/0048-5764_Psychopharmacology_bulletin

Reisberg, B., Ferris, S. H., Franssen, E. H., Shulman, E., Monteiro, I., Sclan, S. G., . . . & Laska, E. (1996). Mortality and temporal course of probable Alzheimer's disease: A 5-year prospective study. *International Psychogeriatrics*, *8*(2), 291–311. Retrieved from http://journals.cambridge.org/action/displayJournal?jid=IPG

Sampson, E. L., Leurent, B., Blanchard, M. R., Jones, L., & King, M. (2013). Survival of people with dementia after unplanned acute hospital admission: A prospective cohort study. *International Journal of Geriatric Psychiatry*, *28*(10), 1015–1022. doi:10.1002/gps.3919

Timmerman, C. (2012). "Just give me the best quality of life questionnaire": The Karnofsky Scale and the history of quality of life measurements in cancer trials. *Chronic Illness*, *9*(3), 179–190. doi:10.1177/1742395312466903

Victoria Hospice Society. (2001). Palliative Performance Scale (PPSv2). Retrieved from http://www.npcrc.org/files/news/palliative_performance_scale_PPSv2.pdf

Wright, J., & Kinzbrunner, B. M. (2011). Predicting prognosis: How to decide when end-of-life care is needed. In B. M. Kinzbrunner & J. S. Policzer (Eds.), *End-of-life care: A practical guide* (pp. 3–36). New York, NY: McGraw-Hill.

7

Hospice Basics: Admission and Ongoing Care

Using established criteria, hospice nurses assess patients for eligibility for hospice services and help patients and families establish goals of care. If hospice care is deemed appropriate, the patient is admitted to hospice services and the appropriate level of care determined through collaboration of the interdisciplinary team with the patient and family. The nurse's assessment and knowledge of hospice levels of care are integral to this process.

After reading this chapter, you will be able to:

- Conduct a hospice admission
- Orient the patient and family to hospice services
- Assess ongoing eligibility for hospice care

THE HOSPICE ADMISSION

Once it is determined that the patient is eligible for hospice services, the admission can take place. On admission, the nurse should review:

- Patient and family goals
- Goals of hospice care
- Services provided by hospice
- Availability of inpatient services

- Fees or co-pays (if not already reviewed by the social worker)
- Process of discharge and/or revocation

The hospice admission is a pivotal experience for the patient and family and sets the tone for future hospice care experiences (Moon, 2016).

The National Hospice and Palliative Care Organization (NHPCO, 2009) has devised a Hospice Admission Care Map (see Figure 7.1) that outlines the following steps of the hospice admission:

- Referral to hospice
- Verification of eligibility requirements
- Certification of terminal illness by attending physician and hospice medical director
- Election of hospice care by patient
- Admission to hospice
  - Initial and comprehensive assessment
  - Interdisciplinary care planning and coordination of services

ORIENTING FAMILIES TO HOSPICE SERVICES

When a patient is admitted to hospice care, the family should be oriented to the types of services that will be provided. Families should be made aware that hospice care includes:

- Durable medical equipment
- Medication related to the terminal illness
- Routine visits from the hospice nurse
- Twenty-four-hour availability of hospice staff
- Care from the interdisciplinary team

Family caregivers should be made aware that respite care is available in an inpatient facility for up to 5 days each month (Centers for Medicare & Medicaid Services, 2015).

Families should also be made aware that hospice care does not encompass:

- Curative treatment of the terminal illness
- Emergency services
- Live-in caretakers
- Long-term inpatient services
- Ongoing individual counseling

ESTABLISHING ONGOING ELIGIBILITY

When a patient is admitted to hospice care, the certification of the terminal illness is considered to be valid for a period of 6 months. Medicare defines this as two 90-day certification periods. After these two 90-days periods, recertification of the terminal illness is required. Patients who continue to meet eligibility requirements can be recertified for an unlimited number of 60-day periods. When documenting a patient's ongoing eligibility for hospice care, the hospice nurse should reference the Local Coverage Determination guidelines and appropriate assessment tools.

FACE-TO-FACE ENCOUNTERS

As a result of the Affordable Care Act, Medicare requires that hospice patients be seen by the hospice nurse practitioner or medical director prior to the third benefit (180 days). The purpose of the face-to-face encounter is to verify continued eligibility for hospice services. The nurse practitioner should work closely with the hospice nurse to review the patient's status and determine ongoing eligibility.

PATIENT DISCHARGE

In instances where the patient is no longer deemed eligible for hospice due to an improvement in health, the patient will be discharged from the service. Patients themselves may also initiate discharge if they seek curative treatment and are no longer amenable to the goals of hospice care. In such cases, the patient will revoke the hospice benefit. When a patient is discharged, a discharge order must be written by the hospice medical director and the hospice team must include the

Patient referred for hospice service.

(§ 418.20 Eligibility requirements; Subpart B)

- Hospice may meet with patient/ family to discuss hospice services.
- Meeting purpose: to discuss hospice care with the patient/family and to establish eligibility for hospice services. *This is not the "initial assessment" visit.*

Each hospice may have a different definition regarding when the patient is "admitted" to hospice care. This map utilizes the language from the Medicare hospice regulations and is only one example of the admission process.

(§418.22 Certification of terminal illness; Subpart B)

✓ Attending physician signs the certificate of terminal illness form.

✓ Hospice medical director signs the certificate of terminal illness form.

- **Related: § 418.102 - Medical director.**

These steps may occur simultaneously

(§418.24 Election of hospice care; Subpart B)

Patient elects hospice care by signing a notice of hospice care election form (NOE). The effective date may be later than the signing date.

This is the first allowable date of billing.

NOTE: Verbal election of the hospice benefit by the patient or representative is not allowable per CMS.

(§ 418.25 Admission to hospice care; Subpart B)

- Hospice admits patient on the recommendation of medical director in consultation with the attending physician (if any).
- The hospice medical director must consider at least the following information:
  - Diagnosis of the terminal condition of the patient.
  - Other health conditions, whether related or unrelated to the terminal condition.
  - Current clinically relevant information supporting all diagnoses.

(§ 418.52 Patient Rights; Subpart C)

The hospice reviews all admission paperwork including the notice of rights in a language and manner that the patient/ family understands. The patient/ representative signs a form indicating that patient rights notice was received.

Additional patient / representative signature documents may include:

- Consent for care
- Financial agreement
- Medicare Secondary paperwork

(§ 418.54 Initial and comprehensive assessment of the patient; Subpart C)

- Hospice interdisciplinary group (IDG) completes comprehensive assessment no later than 5 calendar days after the election of hospice care.
- The IDG consults with the individual's attending physician (if any) and develops individualized patient plan of care from assessed needs.
- Content for the comprehensive assessment is outlined in § 418.54 (c)
- Hospice staff discusses the hospice policies/ procedures for safe use and disposal of controlled drugs with the patient or representative and the family in a language and manner that they understand and documents in the patient's clinical record that information was provided and discussed. (if controlled drugs introduced this visit)

Comprehensive assessment tools and process are the hospice provider's choice.

The effective date of the notice of hospice election is the billing start date.

The "election of hospicecare" is the effective date of the election date of the election statement. The patient may sign the hospice election statement with a later (not earlier) effective date.

(§ 418.54 Initial and comprehensive assessment of the patient; Subpart C)

- The hospice RN must complete an initial assessment within **48 hours** of the **effective date** of the election of hospice care.
- This is an assessment of the patient's/ family's immediate care needs.
- The comprehensive nursing assessment may be completed during this first assessment visit as appropriate.

(§ 418.56 Interdisciplinary group, care planning, and coordination of services; Subpart C)

- The IDG RN coordinates the patient's plan of care.
- The written plan of care is established by the hospice IDG in collaboration with the attending physician (if any), the patient or representative, and the primary caregiver.
- The hospice must ensure that each patient and the primary care giver(s) receive education and training provided by the hospice as appropriate to their responsibilities for the care and services identified in the plan of care.
- The plan of care must include all services necessary for the palliation and management of the terminal illness and related conditions.
- Content for the patient plan of care is outlined in **§ 418.56 (c)**

(§ 418.106 Condition of participation: Drugs and biologicals, medical supplies, and durable medical equipment; Subpart D)

- The interdisciplinary group confers with an individual with education and training in drug management as defined in hospice policies and procedures and State law, who is an employee of or under contract with the hospice to ensure that drugs and biologicals meet each patient's needs.
- The interdisciplinary group, as part of the review of the plan of care, must determine the ability of the patient and/or family to safely self-administer drugs and biologicals to the patient in his or her home.

(§ 418.56 Interdisciplinary group, care planning, and coordination of services)

Review of the plan of care.

- Hospice IDG (in collaboration with the individual's attending physician, if any) must review, revise, and document the individualized plan **as frequently as the patient's condition requires, but no less frequently than every 15 calendar days.**

- Revised plan of care must include information from the patient's updated comprehensive assessment and must note the patient's progress toward outcomes and goals specified in the plan of care.

(§ 418.54 Initial and comprehensive assessment of the patient; Subpart C)

Update of the comprehensive assessment.

- Accomplished by hospice IDG in collaboration with the individual's attending physician, (if any)

- Must consider changes that have taken place since the initial assessment.

- Must include information about patient's progress toward desired outcomes, and a re-assessment of the patient's response to care.

- Assessment update must be accomplished **as frequently as the condition of the patient requires, but no less frequently than every 15 days.**

Resources:

✓ **CoP and interpretive guidelines information, tool, and other resources at NHPCO's Regulatory and Compliance Center at org/regulatory**

✓ **The Centers for Medicare & Medicaid Services Hospice Center at** www.cms.hhs.gov/center/hospice.asp

✓ **Ask NHPCO's Regulatory Assistance a question at** regulatory@nhpco.org

✓

Figure 7.1 NHPCO Hospice Admission Care Map (NHPCO, 2009).

patient and family in the discharge planning process (National Hospice and Palliative Care Organization, 2016).

CONCLUSION

This chapter offered a review of how to determine a patient's eligibility for hospice care based on Local Coverage Determination guidelines. Several tools that are commonly used to document patients' status on an ongoing basis were also discussed. Additionally, the role of the nurse in documenting continued eligibility for hospice care was presented.

References

Centers for Medicare & Medicaid Services. (2015). Medicare benefit policy manual. Retrieved from https://www.cms.gov/Regulations-and-Guidance/Guidance/Manuals/downloads/bp102c09.pdf

Moon, P. J. (2016). Hospice admission assessment: A narrative view. *American Journal of Hospice & Palliative Medicine*. Advance online publication. doi:10.1177/1049909115624375

National Hospice and Palliative Care Organization. (2009). Hospice admission care map. Retrieved from http://www.nhpco.org/sites/default/files/public/regulatory/Hospice_admission_map-2009-F_(2).pdf

National Hospice and Palliative Care Organization. (2016). Discharge from hospice services. Retrieved from http://www.nhpco.org/discharge-hospice-services

8

Levels of Care

When working with patients and families, hospice nurses are often asked to make recommendations for patient care in the home and in other care settings. The focus of this chapter is on the role of the nurse in assessing patients' needs, determining appropriate levels of care, and communicating with other members of the health care team.

After reading this chapter, you will be able to:

- Assess patient care needs to determine the appropriate level of care
- Differentiate the types of hospice care provided at each level of care
- Discuss tools used to structure interprofessional communication during patient transitions

DETERMINING PATIENT NEEDS

Hospice nurses must make recommendations regarding which level of care is most appropriate for a patient and family on admission to service (see Exhibits 8.1 and 8.2). For some patients, home care is the most appropriate level of care because there is a caregiver present and the patient prefers to stay at home rather than transfer to an inpatient facility. In other cases, inpatient care may be most appropriate due to the

Exhibit 8.1

Assessment of the Patient's Goals and Wishes

- What is most important to the patient right now?
- If the patient's condition were to change, would he or she want to stay at home or go to an inpatient setting?
- What symptoms or conditions would make the patient or family consider a hospital admission?
- Does the patient have a living will? Is a POLST order written and accessible?

POLST, Physician Orders for Life-Sustaining Treatment.

Exhibit 8.2

Assessment of Care Needs

- Is there a reliable caregiver in the home?
- Is the home environment safe?
- Can the patient's symptoms be managed at home by the caregiver with the support of the hospice team?
- Is the patient experiencing acute symptoms? Can the symptoms be managed most effectively in an inpatient hospice setting?
- Does the patient already reside in a long-term care facility? Is the staff able to co-manage end-of-life concerns with the hospice team?
- Can the patient's symptoms be managed in the home with continuous care from the hospice staff?

lack of a caregiver or because it is in line with the patient's preferences. The decision-making process for determining the appropriate level of care is complex and involves a series of questions and decisions on the part of the family and the nurse.

After completing the assessment, the nurse, in consultation with the patient, family, and hospice team, recommends the appropriate level of care, which may include:

- **Routine home care:** Care of the hospice patient is provided in the home with regularly scheduled visits from the hospice team.
- **Continuous home care:** Continuous care is provided in the home, predominantly by nurses, but can be supplemented with hospice aides. This type of care is intended to support patients and families through crises on a short-term basis in order to allow the patient to stay at home.

- **Inpatient respite care:** Care is provided within an approved facility for a short period of time to allow respite for the caregiver(s).
- **General inpatient (GIP) care:** Care is provided in an inpatient facility to achieve pain control or symptom management that cannot be accomplished at home (Centers for Medicare & Medicaid Services, 2015a; see Part V for a review of Medicare regulations pertinent to GIP care).
- **Last 7 days:** A change in reimbursement for hospice care took place as of January 1, 2016. This service-intensity-add-on (SIA) was designed to recognize that the care provided for a patient during the last week of life is intense and costly. According to the Centers for Medicare & Medicaid Services (2015b), in order to receive reimbursement in addition to the per diem routine rate, the following criteria must be met:
  - The patient's level of care is "routine home care"
  - The date of care is within the last 7 days of the patient's life
  - Direct patient care is provided by a registered nurse (RN) or licensed social worker

With the appropriate level of care determined, the nurse coordinates the plan of care for the patient. The interdisciplinary team meets regularly (at least every 15 days) to review and revise the plan of care based on the patient's condition and needs (National Hospice and Palliative Care Organization, 2009).

WHEN A PATIENT DIES

As a patient's death draws closer, it is critical for the hospice nurse to maintain close communication with the family members to keep them abreast of any changes in condition and help them to mentally and emotionally prepare for the loss. Family members should be aware that they should call the hospice if they note any changes in the patient's condition, especially if they believe that death has occurred.

Fast Facts in a Nutshell

Laws that govern whether an RN can legally pronounce a patient's death vary from state from state and by practice setting.

Question: How can I determine if RNs can pronounce a death in my state?

Answer: To determine state regulations that govern the practice of an RN in your state visit the National Council of State Boards of Nursing at www.ncsbn.org/npa.htm and use the drop-down menu to find the Nurse Practice Act for your state.

When a call is received that a patient has died at home, the hospice nurse must go to the home to complete an assessment and to support the family. The role of the nurse in pronouncing a patient's death varies from state to state. However, in all states, the nurse is responsible for assessment and family support. When a patient's death occurs, the following steps should be followed (Berry & Griffie, 2015):

- Maintain a calm approach
- Identify the patient
- Assess the patient for breathing, motion, or other signs of life
- Assess for lack of pupillary response, and absent carotid pulses and apical pulses (auscultate for 1 minute in most situations)
- Provide respectful, culturally appropriate post-mortem care

Documentation of the patient's death should include:

- The patient's name
- Time of the call, who called, and who was present at the time of death
- Physical exam findings
- Who made the pronouncement of death, and the time of the pronouncement
- Who was notified of the patient's death
- To whom the patient's body was released

Prior to leaving a patient's home after a death, the nurse disposes of medications using the following recommendations (Nathan & Deamant, 2015):

- Remove medications from their containers, mix with cat litter or used coffee grounds, and place in a plastic bag or tub to prevent diversion.

- When disposing of fentanyl patches, fold the patch in half with the sticky side inward and flush the patch down a toilet.
- Remove labels from patient medication bottles and then throw the empty bottles in the trash or recycle as appropriate.

Additionally, the nurse should document that medications were properly disposed of, following all agency policies and procedures.

Fast Facts in a Nutshell

Effective communication hinges on interdisciplinary collaboration and teamwork (Bhatt & Mitchell, 2015).

COMMUNICATING DURING PATIENT TRANSITIONS

During patient transitions, such as at the time of a patient's death or when a transfer to an inpatient setting from home occurs, the use of a standard communication tool has been recommended to facilitate smooth transitions (The Joint Commission, 2012). One such tool, Situation Background Assessment Recommendation (SBAR), was developed by the military to standardize reports and overcome communication barriers (Pope, Rodzen, & Spross, 2008). SBAR is now widely used in health care settings to convey the following:

- **Situation:** Identify yourself, identify the patient, and succinctly explain what the issue is. In hospice settings, this may also entail information about the patient's home situation and family dynamics.
- **Background:** Provide information that helps to situate the current problem such as pertinent medical history, lab results, and any recent changes in condition.
- **Assessment:** Describe what you think the problem is and the severity of the problem.
- **Recommendation:** Provide a recommendation for what should happen next. This may be the need to prescribe a different prescription drug or change the dosage of currently used medications. Other recommendations may include a change in the level of care, such as a transfer from home to the inpatient unit for symptom management.

CONCLUSION

In this chapter, the hospice nurse's role in determining the appropriate level of care for a patient and coordinating care with the interdisciplinary team during transitions was reviewed. With the information presented in this chapter, the hospice nurse can more effectively establish patient and family needs and organize appropriate care.

References

Berry, P., & Griffie, J. (2015). Preparing for the actual death. In B. R. Ferrell, N. Coyle, & J. A. Paice (Eds.), *Oxford textbook of palliative nursing* (pp. 513–530). New York, NY: Oxford University Press.

Bhatt, A., & Mitchell, A. (2015). Effective collaborative communication in hospice. *Palliative Medicine & Care: Open Access*. Retrieved from http://www.symbiosisonline.org

Centers for Medicare & Medicaid Services. (2015a). Medicare benefit policy manual. Retrieved from https://www.cms.gov/Regulations-and-Guidance/Guidance/Manuals/downloads/bp102c09.pdf

Centers for Medicare & Medicaid Services. (2015b). Hospice payment system. Retrieved from https://www.cms.gov/Outreach-and-Education/Medicare-Learning-Network-MLN/MLNProducts/downloads/hospice_pay_sys_fs.pdf

The Joint Commission. (2012). Transitions of care: The need for a more effective approach to continuing patient care. Retrieved from http://www.jointcommission.org/assets/1/18/hot_topics_transitions_of_care.pdf

Nathan, S., & Deamant, C. D. (2015). Medication disposal #286. *Journal of Palliative Medicine, 18*(1), 82–82. doi:10.1089/jpm.2015.0004

National Hospice and Palliative Care Organization. (2009). Hospice admission care map. Retrieved from http://www.nhpco.org/sites/default/files/public/regulatory/Hospice_admission_map-2009-F_(2).pdf

Pope, B. B., Rodzen, L., & Spross, G. (2008). Raising the SBAR: How better communication improves patient outcomes. *Nursing 2008, 38*(3), 41–43. doi:10.1097/01.NURSE.0000312625.74434.e8

III

End-of-Life Care for Patients and Families

9

Recognizing Existential Suffering and Spiritual Needs and Providing Appropriate Support

In addressing the spiritual needs of patients and families, hospice nurses work closely with the families' spiritual leader, hospice social worker, and hospice chaplain to make sure that the patients' end-of-life wishes are respected and that comforting rituals are implemented. Appropriate assessment of existential suffering ensures that the hospice team can implement interventions to ease patients' suffering.

After reading this chapter, you will be able to:

- Identify symptoms of existential suffering
- Assess patients for signs of spiritual suffering
- Select spiritual assessment tools
- Differentiate between spirituality and religion

EXISTENTIAL SUFFERING

Existential suffering is different from, but may be related to, physical suffering. Existential suffering involves a deep sense of loss, hopelessness, and helplessness that can evolve as one faces the end of life (Kissane, 2012). According to Kissane (2012), some types of existential suffering include:

- Death anxiety related to facing the unknowable
- Loss and change
- Loss of control over choices
- Loss of dignity
- Aloneness
- Poor quality relationship with others
- Feeling that life is meaningless

Fast Facts in a Nutshell

Symptoms of existential distress include: fear, crying, sadness, emotional lability, need for control, isolation, family conflict, loss of faith or spirituality, feelings of hopelessness (Kissane, 2012).

SPIRITUAL SUFFERING

Spiritual suffering is one aspect of existential suffering. Spiritual issues arise at the end of life as patients face the unknown and question what might happen after they take their last breaths. In hospice, nurses work with chaplains, social workers, and other members of the interdisciplinary team to meet patients' and families' spiritual needs. Key skills for hospice nurses include the ability to:

- Assess spiritual suffering
- Meet patients' immediate needs
- Work with other members of the health care team to develop and implement a plan for ongoing support

Fast Facts in a Nutshell

According to The Joint Commission, assessment of spiritual needs is required for every patient.

Tools for assessing spirituality and spiritual distress include:

- FICA Spiritual History Tool© (Puchalski & Romer, 2000)
- FACT Spiritual History Tool (LaRocca-Pitts, 2009)

- The HOPE questions (Anadarajah & Hight, 2001)
- The Spiritual Distress Assessment Tool (Monod et al., 2010)

Question: What is the difference between religion and spirituality?
Answer: Religion is a shared set of beliefs among those who share the same faith tradition. Religions usually include standards of behaviors, rituals, and symbols. Spirituality is the way that individuals express connectedness. Spirituality can be manifested through religion but it can be conveyed without adherence to a particular religion. Spirituality is often individualistically manifested and can take on many forms.

CONCLUSION

Hospice nurses frequently encounter patients who are struggling with religious, spiritual, or existential issues. Knowing how to assess for signs of distress and how to partner with other members of the interdisciplinary team is critical for ensuring the provision of holistic, evidence-based care.

References

Anadarajah, G., & Hight, E. (2001). Spirituality and medical practice: Using the HOPE questions as a practical tool for spiritual assessment. *American Family Physician, 63*, 81–89. Retrieved from http://www.aafp.org/afp

Kissane, D. W. (2012). The relief of existential suffering. *Archives of Internal Medicine, 172*(19), 1501–1505. doi:10.1001/archinternmed.2012.3633

LaRocca-Pitts, M. A. (2009). FACT: Taking a spiritual history in a clinical setting. *Journal of Health Care Chaplaincy, 15*(1), 1–12. doi:10.1080/0885 4720802698350

Monod, S. M., Rochat, E., & Büla, C. J., Jobin, G. Martin, E., & Spencer, B. (2010). The spiritual distress assessment tool: An instrument to assess spiritual distress in hospitalised elderly persons. *BMC Geriatrics, 10*(1), 88. doi:10.1186/1471-2318-10-88

Puchalski, C., & Romer, A. (2000). Taking a spiritual history allows clinicians to understand patients more fully. *Journal of Palliative Medicine, 3*(1), 129–137. doi:10.1089/jpm.2000.3.129

10

Nursing Considerations for Cultural Variations at the End of Life

Religious beliefs and rituals often bring comfort and hope to patients at the end of their lives. Religious and cultural customs are often intertwined and can be manifested by different families in many different ways. Thus, it is crucial to clarify with the patient and family which beliefs and rituals are important and meaningful for them. Likewise, it is important to note that not all individuals who follow a particular religion will accept all of its precepts, so clarifying which aspects of a religion have meaning for each patient is critical in delivering culturally appropriate care. With these caveats noted, this chapter provides an overview of several widely recognized religious traditions, with a particular emphasis on how these religious perspectives may influence patient and family wishes at the end of life.

After reading this chapter, you will be able to:

- Identify how religious traditions can be used to promote comfort for terminally ill patients and their families
- Discuss key points of five major world religions
- Provide examples of common end-of-life practices within various faith traditions

OVERVIEW OF MAJOR WORLD RELIGIONS

Buddhism

The central beliefs of Buddhism are rooted in the enlightened teaching of Siddhartha Gautama and offer instruction on how to free oneself from suffering and live in a state of contentedness (Bruce, 2012). Buddhism is a flexible and moderate religion; its practices are often influenced by and evolve with changing cultural traditions (Bülow et al., 2008). Buddhism teaches:

- Birth and death occur in a cycle.
- Reincarnation does not necessarily mean that one will return in human form. Rather, one may return in any number of living forms.
- The circumstances of one's life and death contribute to the circumstances of one's rebirth. Thus, it is important to create the conditions for a "good death."
  (Bruce, 2012; Webb & Stouffer, 2014)

Creating opportunities for a "good death" entails providing an environment in which the dying person can cultivate a calm mental state even as death approaches (Bruce, 2012; Webb & Stouffer, 2014). Creating a peaceful environment may involve:

- Minimizing interventions
- Lowering lighting
- Playing music that the patient and family find soothing

Fast Facts in a Nutshell

The family may provide an image of the Buddha or create an altar near the patient's bedside and prayers may be said to comfort the patient (Bruce, 2012).

Buddhists believe that after death, it may take several days for one to fully disconnect from the body. Thus, it is best to allow the body to be undisturbed for as long as possible. In the past, some Buddhists were opposed to organ donation because of this belief (Webb & Stouffer,

2014), but these attitudes are shifting, and organ donation is becoming acceptable to some Buddhists (Bülow et al., 2008).

Christianity

Christianity is a religion rooted in the teachings of Jesus Christ, which are contained primarily in the New Testament of the Bible. Like most other religions, Christians can be considered conservative, moderate, or liberal. There are many branches of the Christian faith, including Catholic, Protestant, Orthodox, and independent churches. Often, when patients identify as part of the Christian faith, they will specify a branch such as "Roman Catholic," or state that they are, for example "Methodist" or "Episcopalian," which are branches of Protestantism.

Fast Facts in a Nutshell

Religious rituals, such as the Eucharist (when bread and wine are shared) and baptism (when a person is washed of sins and welcomed into the faith), have their basis in the religious scriptures.

Most Christians incorporate both the Old and New Testaments of the Bible into their spiritual practices, but emphasis is placed on the New Testament, particularly the acts and words of Jesus. The key point in Christianity is the notion that Jesus died and rose from the dead. Based on this critical doctrine, most Christians believe in an afterlife and follow certain tenets of the religion to ensure that they will be acceptable to God at the time of death. Many Christians request special clerical blessings during illness or at the time of death. The practice of confession is common, particularly among Catholics, and involves stating one's sins to a priest and then receiving a blessing of forgiveness. This may be particularly important for patients in the last weeks and days of life. Practices that may be comforting to Christian patients nearing death include:

- Reading sections of the Bible
- Arranging a visit from a patient's spiritual leader, often called a "priest" or "minister"
- Arranging for sacraments such as communion (Eucharist)

Christian families may place religious objects such as crosses, medals, or beads near or on the patient. Holy water or oils may also be used to bless the patient. At the time of death, there is no prohibition against removing these objects from the body. However, these articles should be offered back to the family and never discarded.

Tending to the sick is a key element of the Christian faith; Christians believe that what is done to one who is sick or in need is done to Jesus himself (Soskice, 2012). Therefore, it is very important to provide space and privacy for family members to be involved in care and to be present with their loved ones as death approaches.

Christianity does not include any prescribed rituals for preparing the body; this is left to the preference of the family (Kemp & Bhungalia, 2002). The religion teaches that those who die are in the care of the Lord and extended grief rituals are not largely recognized. In fact, Christians have historically been expected to move on quickly after a loss. However, Western culture has advanced current understandings of grief and mourning and Christian families may increasingly seek counseling or support after the loss of a loved one (Kemp & Bhungalia, 2002).

Hinduism

The term "Hindu" refers to those who are from a specific area in India (Flood, 1996). Many traditions and beliefs are incorporated within Hinduism; it is a religious tradition without rigid doctrine (Rambachan, 2012). Yet, even though there is not one central leader or set of required beliefs, most Hindus are familiar with the religion's foundational texts:

- The Vedas
- The Bhagavad Gita
- The Mahabharata
- The Ramayana
- The Bhagavata Purana

Fast Facts in a Nutshell

Family members may read or chant the teachings of sacred texts in order to calm their loved one and ease the transition through the dying process (Rambachan, 2012).

The sacred texts impart the major tenets of Hinduism including the interconnected concepts of karma and samsara (Rambachan, 2012). To Hindus, the circumstances of the death are critical because they can affect the circumstances of the next life. Death in an intensive care unit or after a prolonged period of artificial support are not considered to be good circumstances for transitioning out of this life (Bülow et al., 2008).

Question: What is the difference between samsara and karma?
Answer: Samsara is the endless cycle of death and rebirth to which all souls are bound. Karma is the belief that one's circumstances in life are related to actions in one's past lives, whether they were good or bad. Just as one's own actions can have an effect on future life circumstances, one's state of mind at the time of transitioning through the process can also have bearing on the next life (Bülow et al., 2008; Rambachan, 2012).

Some Hindus may wear rosary beads, threads, or a red string that is often tied to the wrist. One's body may be marked with symbols that communicate purity or other religious values. At the time of death, no religious objects should be removed from the deceased and no markings should be washed off without permission from the family (Arritt, 2014; Rambachan, 2012).

Islam

Islam is rooted in the teachings of the Prophet Muhammad. Followers of Islam are called Muslims. The Prophet Muhammad is believed to have received his first revelations from God around 610 CE. Muhammad himself shared his revelations verbally, and these teachings were later written and disseminated by his followers in the Qur'an (Lapidus, 2014). The Qur'an makes clear that illness and death are part of God's plan for individuals and are meant to be learning experiences that can spur spiritual growth. Thus, Muslims generally bear suffering with courageous resignation to God's will (Waugh, 2012).

Fast Facts in a Nutshell

The Qur'an is the holy book of Islam and contains the teachings that God revealed to Muhammad.

Muslims believe that those who die belong to God in the afterlife. Thus, facing the end of one's life may prompt introspection and spiritual preparedness. Proper preparation is crucial because Muslims believe that crossing over into the afterlife involves judgment and atonement (Waugh, 2012). Particular rituals may be undertaken and must be supported by the end-of-life care team. For example, devout Muslims pray five times each day and engage in ritual cleansing before prayers. Assisting a patient to do this, even when the patient is nearing death, can be very comforting to the patient and family. When a Muslim patient is nearing death, it may be comforting to:

- Encourage family members to draw near and pray with the patient as desired
- Suspend medical interventions during prayers
- Note dietary restrictions such as avoidance of pork or pork products
- Ensure the availability of halal (meat from animals that have been killed according to religious laws) (Kemp & Bhunghalia, 2002; Waugh, 2012)

It is important to note that modesty is highly regarded among Muslims and same-sex health care providers should provide care whenever possible (Kemp & Bhungalia, 2002). The body should be exposed only when absolutely necessary (Cheraghi, Payne, & Salsali, 2005). At the time of death, the following should be observed:

- The patient's body should be covered at all times.
- The patient's body should be washed and positioned so that his or her feet face the direction of Mecca.
- The family may place a Qur'an near the body, or sometimes may place certain stones or beads on the body (Cheraghi et al., 2005).
- The family should be provided with space, time, and privacy to carry out religious rituals.

Judaism

Judaism is a religion in the Abrahamic tradition, dating back to 1500 to 1000 BCE (Kemp & Bhungalia, 2002). There are three main branches of Judaism:

1. Orthodox Jews strictly follow Jewish laws called "halakha." Orthodox Jews do not write "God"; rather they write "G-d" to avoid profaning the holy name.
2. Conservative Jews also follow Jewish laws but allow for moderation according to cultural and temporal norms.
3. Reform Jews constitute the most liberal branch of Judaism and do not follow a strict interpretation of the halakha. Rather, Reform Jews identify more closely with the moral ideals of the faith (Kemp & Bhungalia, 2002).

Fast Facts in a Nutshell

The sacred text of Judaism is called the Tanakh, which comprises the Torah, Nevi'im, and Ketuvim (Novak, 1994).

At the end of life:

- Jewish patients may request spiritual support and guidance from a Rabbi.
- Time and space should be afforded to the family to remain close to their loved one (Kemp & Bhungalia, 2002).
- Family members may wish to say traditional prayers with their loved one. The Kaddish is a prayer used at the end of life (Kemp & Bhungalia, 2002).
- Withholding food and fluids is not acceptable unless that patient is actively dying and feeding the patient would cause pain or distress (Bülow et al., 2008).
- Preferences for kosher food (food prepared in accordance with religious laws) may be noted and should be accommodated.

After the patient's death:

- The patient's eyes should be closed and the body should remain covered.

- Religious objects should not be removed from the body.
- Facial hair should not be cut or shaved.
- Family members often remain with the patient's body until burial. Some Jewish families also request that nurses refrain from removing tubes and catheters from the body, preferring to allow the funeral director to do this when preparing for burial, which typically takes place within 24 hours of the death.

After the burial, the period of mourning, which is called "Shiva," is observed. During this time, certain restrictions on behavior and social activities are observed (Kemp & Bhungalia, 2002). This may vary according to the family's adherence to Jewish law. Health care providers should clarify the family's preferences prior to offering bereavement visits.

CONCLUSION

When working with diverse populations at the end of life, nurses should promote patient dignity, treat all patients with respect, and help patients face terminal illness by making decisions about the care they would like to receive (Periyakoil, Stevens, & Kraemer, 2013).

References

Arritt, T. (2014). Caring for patients of different religions. *Nursing Made Incredibly Easy*, *12*(6), 38–45. Retrieved from http://journals.lww.com/nursingmadeincrediblyeasy/Pages/default.aspx

Bruce, A. (2012). Welcoming an old friend: Buddhist perspectives on good death. In H. Coward & K. I. Stajduhar (Eds.), *Religious understandings of a good death in hospice palliative care* (pp. 29–50). Albany: State University of New York Press.

Bülow, H. H., Sprung, C. L., Reinhart, K., Prayag, S., Du, B., Armaganidis, A., . . . & Levy, M. M. (2008). The world's major religions' points of view on end-of-life decisions in the intensive care unit. *Intensive Care Medicine*, *34*(3), 423–430. Retrieved from http://icmjournal.esicm.org/index.html

Cheraghi, M. A., Payne, S., & Salsali, M. (2005). Spiritual aspects of end-of-life care for Muslim patients: Experiences from Iran. *International Journal of Palliative Nursing*, *11*, 468–474. Retrieved from http://www.magonlinelibrary.com/toc/ijpn/current

Flood, G. (1996). *An introduction to Hinduism*. New York, NY: Cambridge University Press.

Kemp, C., & Bhungalia, S. (2002). Culture and the end of life: A review of major world religions. *Journal of Hospice & Palliative Nursing*, 4(4), 235–242. Retrieved from http://lww.com/jhpn/toc/2002/10000/Culture_and_the_End_of_Life__A_Review_of_Major.22.aspx

Lapidus, I. M. (2014). *A history of Islamic societies*. Cambridge, UK: Cambridge University Press.

Novak, P. (1994). *The world's wisdom*. San Francisco, CA: HarperCollins.

Periyakoil, V. S., Stevens, M., & Kraemer, H. (2013). Multicultural long-term care nurses' perceptions of factors influencing patient dignity at the end of life. *Journal of the American Geriatric Society*, 61, 440–446. doi:10.1111/jgs.12145

Rambachan, A. (2012). "Like a ripe fruit separating from a vine": Religious understandings of a good death: Hinduism. In H. Coward & K. I. Stajduhar (Eds.), *Religious understandings of a good death in hospice palliative care* (pp. 29–50). Albany: State University of New York Press.

Soskice, J. (2012). "Dying well in Christianity": Religious understandings of a good death: Hinduism. In H. Coward & K. I. Stajduhar (Eds.), *Religious understandings of a good death in hospice palliative care* (pp. 29–50). Albany: State University of New York Press.

Waugh, E. (2012). Muslim perspectives on a good death in hospice and end-of-life care. In H. Coward & K. I. Stajduhar (Eds.), *Religious understandings of a good death in hospice palliative care* (pp. 77–98). Albany: State University of New York Press.

Webb, J., & Stouffer, L. E. (2014). Religious and spiritual differences within families: Influences on end-of-life decision making. *The Journal for Nurse Practitioners*, 10(8), 588–593. Retrieved from http://www.npjournal.org

11

Assessing and Responding to Physical Changes and Symptoms at the End of Life

Although each person's death is as unique as the life lived, there are symptoms that hospice nurses assess and treat regularly. This chapter discusses common end-of-life symptoms along with palliative nursing interventions. Medications that are commonly used to treat these symptoms are also presented.

After reading this chapter, you will be able to:

- Identify common end-of-life symptoms
- Discuss appropriate nursing interventions used to treat end-of-life symptoms
- Name medications used to treat end-of-life symptoms

COMMON END-OF-LIFE SYMPTOMS

Anxiety

Anxiety often occurs at the end of life as patients experience a lack of control over their own health and face their own deaths. Anxiety often manifests as agitation, inability to sleep, irritability, and inability to focus (see Exhibit 11.1).

Exhibit 11.1

Interventions for Anxiety

Nursing interventions
- Offer therapeutic presence and therapeutic touch
- Play soothing music
- Teach deep breathing and relaxation exercises
- Assure quality care until life's end
- Collaborate with members of the interdisciplinary team to help identify and treat the cause of the anxiety

Pharmacologic treatment options
- Antidepressant therapy (if depressive symptoms coexist)
- Benzodiazepines (e.g., lorazepam, temazepam)
- Barbiturates (e.g., pentobarbital, thioridazine)

Source: Kinzbrunner, Wright, Schlecter, and Maluso-Bolton (2011).

Edema

Lower extremity edema can occur at the end of life due to chronic conditions such as heart failure or liver disease. Other causes such as immobility, metastasis, and blood clots can also lead to peripheral edema (Kinzbrunner & Wright, 2011). Edema can cause discomfort, weakness, and decreased mobility. Edema that arises at the end of life is often refractory (see Exhibit 11.2).

Exhibit 11.2

Interventions for Edema

Nursing interventions
- Elevation of lower extremities
- Excellent skin care
- Limit salt intake

Pharmacologic treatment options
- Diuretics
- Albumin (IV)

Source: Kinzbrunner and Wright (2011).

Constipation

Constipation is a common symptom at the end of life that may be caused or exacerbated by medications (especially opioids), decreased fluid intake, and immobility. Neurological diseases and spinal cord injuries may also contribute to constipation. Bowel obstruction secondary to adhesions or tumors can also cause an inability to pass stool (Kinzbrunner & McInnis, 2011; see Exhibit 11.3).

Exhibit 11.3

Interventions for Constipation

Nursing interventions
- Encourage fluid intake
- Schedule toileting
- Increase mobility as tolerated
- Increase fiber intake as tolerated
- Monitor for loose stools or diarrhea that may be a sign of a fecal impaction
- Carefully document bowel regimen
- Administer stool softeners routinely (not prn) for patients on opioid medications
- Digitally disimpact if necessary (patient should be premedicated for pain/anxiety)

Pharmacologic treatment options
- Polyethylene glycol 3350
- Docusate sodium
- Senna/docusate sodium
- Bisacodyl (po or suppository PR)
- Fleet enema
- Lactulose

Sources: Hellsten and Berg (2015); Kinzbrunner and McInnis (2011).

Delirium

Delirium typically has an acute onset and involves "impaired attention, altered awareness, and a variety of cognitive and neuropsychiatric disturbances" (Adamis, Devaney, Shanahan, McCarthy, & Meagher, 2015, p. 1). Delirium that occurs around the time of death is often called "terminal agitation" and may include fearfulness and hallucinations (Heidrich & English, 2015). Early intervention is necessary to reverse symptoms of delirium, if possible. In rare cases, palliative sedation may be considered as a last resort (Kinzbrunner, Wright, Schlecter, & Maluso-Bolton, 2011; see Exhibit 11.4).

Exhibit 11.4

Interventions for Delirium

Nursing interventions
- Provide a therapeutic environment
- Provide music therapy
- Promote activity as tolerated
- Seek the cause (e.g., constipation, fatigue, medication reactions, hypoxia, pain)
- Avoid use of restraints

Pharmacologic treatment options
- Haloperidol
- Chlorpromazine
- Risperidone
- Lorazepam

Sources: Heidrich and English (2015); Kinzbrunner, Wright, Schlecter, & Maluso-Bolton (2011).

Dyspnea

Dyspnea is a subjective experience of breathlessness. Although many disease processes contribute to dyspnea, especially diseases of the heart and lungs, it can occur at the end of life for many reasons. For example, fluid imbalance, immobility, neurological disease, and tumors can contribute to dyspnea. When possible, the cause of dyspnea should be identified and corrected. Regardless of the root cause, palliation of dyspnea is critical at the end of life to promote comfort (see Exhibit 11.5).

Exhibit 11.5

Interventions for Dyspnea

Nursing interventions
- Careful assessment of dyspnea
- Determination of factors that worsen or improve dyspnea
- Assessment of signs of poor perfusion such as cyanosis
- Repositioning
- Use of fans (or moving air)

Pharmacologic treatment options
- Opioids (oral or systemic)
- Bronchodilators

(continued)

Exhibit 11.5

Interventions for Dyspnea *(continued)*

- Corticosteroids
- Anxiolytics
- Oxygen (this is most beneficial for patients who are hypoxic)

Sources: Dudgeon (2015); Negron and McInnis (2011).

Nausea and Vomiting

Nausea and vomiting may occur at the end of life due to treatments such as chemotherapy, neurological disease, and tumors. Patients may suffer from lack of appetite, anxiety, insomnia, and pain due to nausea and vomiting. Aspiration is also a concern for some patients (see Exhibit 11.6).

Exhibit 11.6

Interventions for Nausea and Vomiting

Nursing interventions
- Reduce or remove sights, sounds, and smells that trigger nausea
- Treat underlying causes of nausea/vomiting, if possible
- Assess for constipation and fecal impaction
- Provide small, frequent meals; offer foods according to patient's preference

Pharmacologic treatment options
- Prochlorperazine or chlorpromazine
- Metoclopramide
- Dexamethasone
- Haloperidol
- Hydroxyzine
- Scopolamine

Sources: Chow, Cogan, and Mun (2015); Kinzbrunner and McInnis (2011).

Pain

Physical pain is a very common symptom at the end of life and is often related to disease processes. Pain is distressing to both the patient and the family. It is roundly considered the only emergency in hospice care and as such should be treated promptly. Thus, careful assessment of

P: Palliative and provocative factors

Ask: What makes the pain better or worse?

- The patient's response to this question helps the nurse to determine whether the pain regimen is effective or needs to be modified according to the patient's report.

Q: Quality of the pain

Ask: Can you describe what the pain feels like to you?

- The words the patient uses to describe the pain help the nurse to differentiate what type of pain the patient is experiencing.
- "Neuropathic pain" is generally described as burning, tingling, shocking, shooting, radiating, numbness, "pins and needles."
- "Visceral pain" is generally described as gnawing, stretching, pressure, crampy, deep, poorly localized.
- "Somatic pain" is generally described as dull, sore, throbbing.

R: Radiation

Ask: Is the pain in one area? Can you point to it? Does it travel or radiate?

- The response to these questions helps to differentiate neuropathic from somatic pain or visceral pain.
- Pain that is well-localized is generally somatic. Pain that radiates is usually neuropathic. Visceral pain is often poorly localized.

S: Severity

Ask: Can you tell me how bad the pain is on a scale of 1 to 10? One means the pain is barely noticeable and 10 means it is the worst pain you have ever felt.

- The patient's response to this question provides a snapshot of how intense the pain is for the patient right now. It also helps the patient and nurse determine if goals are met after intervention.

T: Timing

Ask: Does the pain seem to be better or worse at a certain time of the day? When did it start? How long does it last? Does it ever wake you up?

- The patient's response to these questions helps determine whether the pain is due to muscle fatigue, arthritis, or immobility. It is also useful in planning the timing of interventions to alleveiate the pain.

Figure 11.1 Pain assessment.

pain is crucial. Thorough assessment of pain includes asking patients to describe the pain using the PQRST mnemonic and appropriate interpretation of responses. (See Figure 11.1.)

Once a thorough assessment of the pain is completed, the hospice nurse designs and implements appropriate interventions, monitors the effectiveness of the interventions, and modifies the plan as needed (see Exhibit 11.7).

Exhibit 11.7

Interventions for Pain

Nursing interventions
- Reposition patient for comfort
- Apply heat or cold
- Teach meditation/relaxation techniques
- Massage

Pharmacologic treatment options
- Nonopioids such as acetaminophen, aspirin, ibuprofen, naproxen, choline, magnesium, indomethacin, ketorolac, celecoxib
- Opioids (oral, topical, subcutaneous, IV) such as morphine, fentanyl, oxycodone, methadone, hydromorphone, oxymorphone (*Note:* A laxative should be added to the medication regimen for all patients using opioids.)
- Coanalgesics such as antidepressants, anticonvulsants, corticosteroids, local anesthetics

Sources: Friedman, Kinzbrunner, Weinred, and Clark (2011); Paice (2015).

Terminal Secretions (Death Rattle)

Terminal secretions, also called "terminal congestion," occur frequently at the end of life. They are manifested by a noisy "rattling" sound when the patient breathes. Death rattle is not thought to cause distress to the patient. However, it can be distressing to family members and caregivers (Lokker, van Zuylen, van der Rijt, & van der Heide, 2014; see Exhibit 11.8).

Exhibit 11.8

Interventions for Terminal Secretions

Nursing interventions
- Repositioning
- Oropharyngeal suctioning if necessary (deep suctioning is not recommended)

Pharmacologic treatment options
- Hyoscyamine
- Atropine
- Glycopyrrolate
- Scopolamine

Sources: Dudgeon (2015); Kinzbrunner, Nguyen, and Ash (2011).

CONCLUSION

At the end of life, patients experience a variety of symptoms that may or may not follow a predictable pattern. The goal of care for terminally ill patients is to promote comfort by managing symptoms using pharmacological and/or nonpharmacological interventions. Nursing assessments and interventions are critical for the provision of quality end-of-life care as death approaches.

References

Adamis, D., Devaney, A., Shanahan, E., McCarthy, G., & Meagher, D. (2015). Defining "recovery" for delirium research: A systematic review. *Age and Aging, 44*(2), 318–321. doi:10.1093/ageing/afu152.

Chow, K., Cogan, D., & Mun, S. (2015). Nausea and vomiting. In B. R. Ferrell, N. Coyle, & J. A. Paice (Eds.), *Oxford textbook of palliative nursing* (pp. 176–190). New York, NY: Oxford University Press.

Dudgeon, D. (2015). Dyspnea, terminal secretions, and cough. In B. R. Ferrell, N. Coyle, & J. A. Paice (Eds.), *Oxford textbook of palliative nursing* (pp. 247–261). New York, NY: Oxford University Press.

Friedman, T. C., Kinzbrunner, B. M., Weinred, N. J., & Clark, M. (2011). Dyspnea and other respiratory symptoms. In B. M. Kinzbrunner & J. S. Policzer (Eds.), *End-of-life care: A practical guide* (pp. 191–210). New York, NY: McGraw-Hill.

Heidrich, D. E., & English, N. K. (2015). Delirium, confusion, agitation, and restlessness. In B. R. Ferrell, N. Coyle, & J. A. Paice (Eds.), *Oxford textbook of palliative nursing* (pp. 385–403). New York, NY: Oxford University Press.

Hellsten, M. B., & Berg, S. (2015). Symptom management in pediatric palliative care. In B. R. Ferrell, N. Coyle, & J. A. Paice (Eds.), *Oxford textbook of palliative nursing* (pp. 837–850). New York, NY: Oxford University Press.

Kinzbrunner, B. M., & McInnis, E. A. (2011). Gastrointestinal symptoms near the end of life. In B. M. Kinzbrunner & J. S. Policzer (Eds.), *End-of-life care: A practical guide* (pp. 211–241). New York, NY: McGraw-Hill.

Kinzbrunner, B. M., Nguyen, V. D., & Ash, J. M. (2011). The last days: The actively dying patient. In B. M. Kinzbrunner & J. S. Policzer (Eds.), *End-of-life care: A practical guide* (pp. 309–330). New York, NY: McGraw-Hill.

Kinzbrunner, B. M., & Wright, J. B. (2011). Other common symptoms near the end of life. In B. M. Kinzbrunner & J. S. Policzer (Eds.), *End-of-life care: A practical guide* (pp. 331–347). New York, NY: McGraw-Hill.

Kinzbrunner, B. M., Wright, J. B., Schlecter, B., & Maluso-Bolton, T. (2011). Delirium, depression, and anxiety. In B. M. Kinzbrunner & J. S. Policzer (Eds.), *End-of-life care: A practical guide* (pp. 261–282). New York, NY: McGraw-Hill.

Lokker, M. E., van Zuylen, L., van der Rijt, C. C. D., & van der Heide, A. (2014). Prevalence, impact, & treatment of death rattle: A systematic review. *Journal of Pain & Symptom Management*, *47*(1), 105–122. Retrieved from http://www.jpsmjournal.com

Negron, F. J., & McInnis, E. A. (2011). Dyspnea and other respiratory symptoms. In B. M. Kinzbrunner & J. S. Policzer (Eds.), *End-of-life care: A practical guide* (pp. 191–210). New York, NY: McGraw-Hill.

Paice, J. A. (2015). Pain at the end of life. In B. R. Ferrell, N. Coyle, & J. A. Paice (Eds.), *Oxford textbook of palliative nursing* (pp. 135–153). New York, NY: Oxford University Press.

12

Supporting Family Members and Caregivers

L osing a loved one is one of the most difficult experiences in life. Family members are not always prepared to serve as primary caregivers or to address the symptoms that occur throughout the dying process while also coping with the emotional burden of losing a loved one. This chapter addresses the needs of family members.

After reading this chapter, you will be able to:

- Help families identify signs of approaching death
- Determine teaching needs of families of patients who are actively dying
- Describe supportive interventions for families of patients who are actively dying

In the last days and hours of life, patients experience physical, psychosocial, and spiritual changes that indicate approaching death. These changes should be assessed frequently and documented regularly. Signs of approaching death include:

- Decreased desire for food and fluids
- Increased sleep leading to unresponsiveness
- Confusion
- Cyanosis of extremities

- Terminal secretions (death rattle)
- Visions or dreams of loved ones who have already died
  (Kehl & Kowalkowski, 2012; Kerr et al., 2014)

Fast Facts in a Nutshell

When educating families on what to expect throughout the dying process, it is often helpful to provide written materials or online resources. An excellent resource is available at www.celtichealthcare .com/wp-content/uploads/2013/12/Hospice-Preparing-for -Approaching-Death.pdf.

Families providing care for dying patients often need support and teaching regarding the signs of approaching death. Common symptoms, such as decreased appetite and increased sleeping, can be very distressing to families. Because the family and the patient are the unit of care in hospice, nurses should clearly explain changes as they occur and teach families the meaning of these changes.

When a patient experiences distressing symptoms, it is stressful for the caregivers. The caregivers' responses to these changes should be carefully assessed and addressed. Patient symptoms that are most distressing to family caregivers include:

- Pain
- Lack of appetite
- Weight loss
- Worrying
- Sadness
- Irritability
- Insomnia
  (Ratkowski, Washington, Craig, & Albright, 2015)

Providing around-the-clock care for a terminally ill loved one is challenging because caregivers are often untrained in providing care and assessing and managing symptoms. Faced with the impending loss of a loved one while also managing physical care, caregivers may experience feelings of uncertainty and grief (D'Antonio, 2014).

According to The Cleveland Clinic Foundation (2012), signs of caregiver fatigue can mimic depression and may include:

- Social withdrawal
- Changes in appetite
- Feelings of hopelessness and helplessness
- Irritability
- Frequent illness
- Feelings of wanting to harm self or others

If a caregiver is manifesting signs of caregiver fatigue/caregiver burnout, the hospice nurse should work closely with all members of the interdisciplinary team, especially the social worker and chaplain, to make plans for the provision of appropriate support.

Cloyes et al. (2014) noted in a recent study that caregivers feel most supported by hospice nurses when nurses:

- Affirm the primacy of the caregiver's role
- Consistently impart accurate and useful information about hospice services, specific skills or interventions, and the role of the interdisciplinary team
- Establish a trusting relationship with the caregiver
- Demonstrate respect for the caregiver's knowledge about the patient's preferences and the patient's condition

In addition to actively providing support for the patient and caregiver(s), and working closely with the interdisciplinary team, the hospice nurse should determine if respite care is appropriate to provide the caregiver with some time to rejuvenate. Some families may also consider hiring privately paid caregivers to ease the burden of providing care on their own. As in any other setting, if the hospice nurse suspects that the stress of caregiving is leading to abuse, appropriate actions must be taken.

CONCLUSION

Those caring for a loved one who is approaching death require accurate information about rapidly changing symptoms and appropriate interventions. The emotional and physical toll of providing continuous care for a loved one can lead to caregiver fatigue or burnout. The hospice nurse cares for the patient and a family as a unit and is responsible for assessing the support needs of family caregivers and collaborating with the interdisciplinary team to implement appropriate support measures.

References

The Cleveland Clinic Foundation. (2012). Caregiving: Recognizing burnout. Retrieved from http://my.clevelandclinic.org/health/diseases_conditions/hic_Alzheimers_and_Dementia_Overview/hic_Alzheimers_Disease_The_Role_of_the_Caregiver/hic_Caregiving_Recognizing_Burnout

Cloyes, K. G., Carpenter, J. G., Berry, P. H., Reblin, M., Clayton, M., & Ellington, L. (2014). "A true human interaction": Comparison of family caregiver and hospice nurse perspectives on needs of family hospice caregivers. *Journal of Hospice & Palliative Nursing, 16*(5), 282–290. doi:10.1097/NJH.0000000000000066

D'Antonio, J. (2014). Caregiver grief and anticipatory mourning. *Journal of Hospice & Palliative Nursing, 16*(2), 99–104. doi:10.1097/NJH.0000000000000027

Kehl, K., & Kowalkowski, J. A. (2012). A systematic review of the prevalence of signs of impending death and symptoms in the last 2 weeks of life. *American Journal of Hospice & Palliative Medicine, 30*(6), 601–616. doi:10.1177/1049909112468222

Kerr, C. W., Donnelly, J. P., Wright, S. T. Kuszczak, S. M., Banas, A., Grant, P. C., & Luczkiewicz, D. L. (2014). End-of-life dreams and visions: A longitudinal study of hospice patients' experiences. *Journal of Palliative Medicine, 17*(3), 296–303. doi:10.1089/jpm.2013.0371

Ratkowski, K. L., Washington, K. T., Craig, K. W., & Albright, D. L. (2015). The stress of sadness: The most stressful symptoms for hospice family caregivers. *American Journal of Hospice & Palliative Care, 32*(7), 745–749. doi:10.1177/1049909114540034

13

Understanding Grief and Bereavement

Hospice nurses work with families and caregivers throughout a patient's last months, weeks, and days. During those times, the hospice nurse provides guidance and support as each new symptom appears and the patient draws closer to death. The purpose of this chapter is to provide information about the processes of grief and bereavement for nurses working with grieving families.

After reading this chapter, you will be able to:

- Identify current grief theories
- Discuss the role of the hospice nurse in providing grief support
- Describe red flags that necessitate grief intervention

GRIEF THEORIES

Hospice nurses regularly work with grieving families. Yet, most nursing programs do not include content specifically on grief support. In this section, several current grief theories, models, and concepts are reviewed.

- **Theory of chronic sorrow:** This theory indicates that after a loss, bereaved individuals experience "periods of happiness . . .

interspersed with episodes of re-grief" (Eakes, Burke, & Hainsworth, 1998, p. 180). This theory differs from Parkes's work in that it applies to many situations, not to bereavement only, and is ongoing and cyclical in nature.

- **Grief to personal growth theory:** This theory (Hogan & DeSantis, 1996) states that grief results in various negative emotions but ultimately leads to personal growth, which involves feeling more compassionate, more loving, and more appreciative of one's life and loved ones.

- **Continuing bonds:** This concept denotes the ongoing relationship that bereaved individuals have with their loved ones after the death. Specifically, bereaved individuals may indicate that, although they have moved forward emotionally, their deceased loved one continues to hold a place of value in their lives (Hogan & DeSantis, 1996; Silverman, Nickman, & Worden, 1992).

- **Complicated grief:** This term is used to describe very severe grief symptoms that do not abate over time as expected. Signs include excessive longing; yearning; preoccupation with the deceased; hallucinations; ongoing, intrusive thoughts of the deceased or the circumstances of the loss; and failure to adapt to the loss over time (Horowitz et al., 2003; Prigerson et al., 1996; Shear, 2015; Worden, 1991).

> **Question:** Why isn't Elisabeth Kübler-Ross's work included in the list of grief theorists?
>
> **Answer:** The five stages in Kübler-Ross's model refer to how a person responds when facing his or her *own* death, not to how a person responds to the loss of a loved one.

PROVIDING GRIEF SUPPORT

Grief occurs repeatedly during the illness of a loved one. With each further decline, the family members or caregivers come closer to facing the reality of loss. Hospice nurses provide emotional support as grief emerges and reemerges. Other members of the interdisciplinary team, especially the social worker and chaplain, also offer invaluable support to families as they grieve. The nurse's grief assessment should include:

- Sources of support
- Sources of strength and comfort
- How the family has faced difficulties or losses in the past

Fast Facts in a Nutshell

Quite often, the words "grief" and "bereavement" are used interchangeably but they are not the same thing. The Oxford English Dictionary (2016) offers the following distinction:

Grief: Hardship, suffering, hurt, harm, mental pain, distress, or sorrow.
Bereavement: The fact or state of being bereaved or deprived of anything.

Grief support interventions include:

- Active listening
- Therapeutic presence and silence
- Therapeutic touch
- Providing accurate information about grief and coping
  (Eakes & Hainsworth, 1998)

BEREAVEMENT PLANNING AND FOLLOW-UP

The hospice nurse works with the social worker and chaplain to actively engage family members preparing for the loss of a loved one. Facilitating keepsake projects such as making a quilt with the loved one's clothes, making plaster molds of the loved one's hands, or making a scrapbook may be helpful. Bereavement involves:

- Waves of sorrow that are sometimes very intense
- Intrusive thoughts of the deceased and the circumstances of the death
- Physical symptoms such as loss of appetite, fatigue with inability to sleep well, nausea, and somatic pain
  (Eakes & Hainesworth, 1998; Hogan, Greenfield, & Schmidt, 2001; Parkes, 1971, 1998; Wright, 2016)

The nurse should avoid well-meaning but harmful statements such as:

- "God won't give you more than you can handle."
- "There is a reason for everything."
- "Try to think about the good times."
  (Wright, 2016)

Fast Facts in a Nutshell

According to the Centers for Medicare & Medicaid Services (2015), a Medicare-certified hospice must provide bereavement counseling for 1 year after the patient's death.

When the hospice nurse provides a bereavement call or visit, it should be carefully documented. The hospice nurse should be aware of signs of complicated grief and if signs of problematic coping are noted, the interdisciplinary team should be notified promptly so that the treatment plan can be modified. Red flags include:

- Prolonged inability to carry out activities of daily living
- Excessive preoccupation with the deceased
- Denial of the loss or inability to accept that the loss has occurred
- Thoughts of harming oneself or others

CONCLUSION

Hospice nurses frequently encounter grieving and bereaved families when providing care for terminally ill patients. This chapter offered an overview of several grief models and theories that can help frame support interventions. Specific nursing interventions were provided as well as recommendations for when referrals should be made.

References

Centers for Medicare & Medicaid Services. (2015). Medicare benefit policy manual. Retrieved from https://www.cms.gov/Regulations-and-Guidance/Guidance/Manuals/downloads/bp102c09.pdf

Eakes, G. G., Burke, M. L., & Hainsworth, M. A. (1998). Middle-range theory of chronic sorrow. Image: The Journal of Nursing Scholarship, 30(2), 179–184.

Retrieved from http://onlinelibrary.wiley.com/journal/10.1111/(ISSN) 1547-5069

Hogan, N. S., & DeSantis, L. (1996). Basic constructs of a theory of adolescent sibling bereavement. In D. Klass, P. Silverman, & S. Nickman (Eds.), *Continuing bonds: New understandings of grief* (pp. 235–254). Washington, DC: Taylor & Francis.

Hogan, N. S., Greenfield, D. B., & Schmidt, L. A. (2001). Development and validation of the Hogan grief reaction checklist. *Death Studies, 25*(1), 1–32. Retrieved from http://www.tandfonline.com/loi/udst20#.V5urevkrJD8

Horowitz, M. J., Siegel, B., Holen, A., Bonanno, G. A., Milbrath, C., & Stinson, C. H. (2003). Diagnostic criteria for complicated grief disorders. *Focus: The Journal of Lifelong Learning in Psychiatry, 1*, 290–298. doi:10.1176/foc.1.3.290

Oxford English Dictionary. (2016). Bereavement. Retrieved from http://www.oed.com

Parkes, C. M. (1971). *Bereavement: Studies of grief in adult life* (1st ed.). Madison, CT: International Universities Press.

Parkes, C. M. (1998). *Bereavement: Studies of grief in adult life* (3rd ed.). Madison, CT: International Universities Press.

Prigerson, H. G., Bierhals, A. J., Kasl, S. V., Reynolds, C. F., III, Shear, M. K., Newsom, J. T., & Jacobs, S. (1996). Complicated grief as a disorder distinct from bereavement-related depression and anxiety: A replication study. *American Journal of Psychiatry, 153*, 1484–1486. doi:10.1176/ajp.153.11.1484

Shear, M. K. (2015). Complicated grief. *New England Journal of Medicine, 372*, 153–160. doi:10.1056/NEJMcp1315618

Silverman, P. R., Nickman, S. L., & Worden, J. W. (1992). Detachment revisited: The child's reconstruction of a dead parent. *American Journal of Orthopsychiatry, 62*(4), 494–503. Retrieved from http://www.apa.org/pubs/journals/ort

Worden, J. W. (1991). *Grief counselling and grief therapy: A handbook for the mental health practitioner* (2nd ed.). New York, NY: Routledge.

Wright, P. M. (2016). The pushing on theory of maternal perinatal bereavement. In B. P. Black, P. M. Wright, & R. Limbo (Eds.), *Perinatal and pediatric bereavement in nursing and other health professions* (pp. 71–91). New York, NY: Springer Publishing.

IV

Ensuring Quality Care in Hospice

14

Defining Quality in Hospice

Hospice care in the United States has evolved rapidly over the past several decades. What began as a grass-roots movement to improve care of the dying soon became more and more uniform as best practices emerged and standardization of care became the norm. Numerous initiatives have led to the development of a framework of the essential components of hospice and palliative care, which later became the platform for reliable quality measures.

After reading this chapter, you will be able to:

- Discuss the evolution of quality initiatives in end-of-life care
- Define quality of care in the hospice setting
- Identify quality indicators for hospice care

DEFINING QUALITY

The Institute of Medicine (IOM) defined quality in care as "The degree to which health services for individuals and populations increase the likelihood of desired health outcomes and are consistent with current professional knowledge" (IOM, 2001). The IOM then established aims for quality care in the 21st century, noting that it should be:

- Safe
- Effective
- Patient-centered

- Timely
- Efficient
- Equitable

The aims developed by the IOM (2001) served as a call to action for health professionals in all settings. In hospice and palliative care, the National Consensus Project (NCP) was underway, leading to the release of a report regarding the provision of high-quality end-of-life care.

Fast Facts in a Nutshell

"The overall experience of end-of-life care is often assessed after the death using a questionnaire addressed to family members or close friends who have first-hand experience of the end-of-life care provided" (Merriman, 2011, p. 106).

THE NCP

In 2001, the NCP was undertaken by a group of interprofessional palliative care experts who were dedicated to defining the domains of hospice and palliative care, as well as establishing guidelines for this specialty area. In 2004, this group released the landmark document *Clinical Practice Guidelines for Quality Palliative Care*. The eight domains of palliative care identified in the Clinical Practice Guidelines are as follows (Dahlin, 2013):

1. **Structure and Processes of Care:** Describes the composition and qualifications of the interdisciplinary team and defines how the team should collaborate with patients and families.
2. **Physical Aspects of Care:** Emphasizes the management of physical symptoms such as pain, fatigue, anxiety, and others.
3. **Psychological and Psychiatric Aspects of Care:** Defines assessment of the psychosocial needs of patients and families. The requirement for bereavement support is included in this domain.
4. **Social Aspects of Care:** Focuses on leveraging family strengths and social support mechanisms to alleviate family stress.

5. **Spiritual, Religious, and Existential Aspects of Care:** Emphasizes the role of all members of the interdisciplinary team, especially the chaplain, in recognizing and addressing spiritual and existential distress. Specifically, the competency among all team members in understanding and supporting religious practice preferences of patients and families is stressed.
6. **Cultural Aspects of Care:** Describes cultural competence and defines processes for the provision of culturally sensitive care.
7. **Care of the Patient at the End of Life:** Highlights the importance of providing multidimensional interdisciplinary end-of-life care for patients and their families, which includes educating them and guiding them through the dying process.
8. **Ethical and Legal Aspects of Care:** Addresses advance care planning, ethics, and legal aspects of care. The role of the interdisciplinary team in broaching end-of-life conversations and documenting patients' preferences is stressed. Consultation with ethics committees and legal counsel is also emphasized.

The report from the NCP provided the first coherent account of what quality end-of-life care entailed. The *Clinical Practice Guidelines* were endorsed by the National Quality Forum (NQF) in 2006, lending further credence to this excellent work. The Clinical Practice Guidelines underpinned the provision of high-quality, uniform, end-of-life care across multiple practice settings and served as the foundation for many other hospice and palliative care initiatives and guidelines (Dahlin, 2015).

DEVELOPMENT OF HOSPICE GUIDELINES

In 2006, the NQF developed *A National Framework and Preferred Practices for Palliative and Hospice Care Quality: A Consensus Report* based on the guidelines in an effort to improve end-of-life care across the six dimensions of care outlined by the IOM (2001). This report outlined 38 preferred practices for hospice and palliative care programs, in an effort to "provide a supporting structure for the future identification, organization, and endorsement of national voluntary consensus standards that will provide the necessary data for consumers, purchasers, and healthcare professionals to make informed decisions and to improve quality of care" (NQF, 2006, p. 4).

Fast Facts in a Nutshell

Measurement of quality helps ensure the accountability of health care providers (Merriman, 2011).

Gathering data to help determine whether the care provided by a hospice organization aligned with preferred practices helps patients, families, and health care professionals monitor the effectiveness of hospice services using concrete data. The NQF (2006) noted that to be meaningful, data must be gathered at the patient/family level, the organizational or programmatic level, and the system level and must be tied to specific outcomes. Outcomes in hospice and palliative care should (NQF, 2006):

■ Align with one of the quality aims endorsed by NQF
■ Clearly impact one of the quality aims endorsed by NQF
■ Address the unique needs of patients and families facing end-of-life circumstances

Measuring Outcomes

Data in isolation do not help hospice professionals make decisions regarding effectiveness of care. Rather, data from a particular hospice should be compared with data from other hospices to help establish best practices and set benchmarks. Each of the aspects of care that will be monitored must be clearly defined and measureable. Quality measures are precise statements that quantify specific aspects of care. In 2012, NQF endorsed these 14 quality measures on palliative and end-of-life care (NQF, 2012):

■ Pain screening
■ Pain assessment
■ Patients treated with an opioid who are given a bowel regimen
■ Patients with advanced cancer assessed for pain at outpatient visits
■ Dyspnea treatment
■ Dyspnea screening
■ Patients admitted to the ICU who have care preferences documented
■ Treatment preferences

- Percentage of hospice patients with documentation in the clinical record of a discussion of spiritual/religious concerns or documentation that the patient/caregiver did not want to discuss
- Comfortable dying
- Hospitalized patients who die an unexpected death with an implantable cardioverter defibrillator (ICD) that has been deactivated
- Family evaluation of hospice care
- CARE—Consumer Assessment and Reports of End of Life
- Bereaved family survey

The measures endorsed by the NQF provided a platform for the development of quality indicators for hospice and palliative care, which was critical, because in 2010 the Patient Protection and Affordable Care Act (ACA) mandated data collection for hospices. Several key areas of care are now routinely monitored and the data can be used for quality monitoring, benchmarking, and comparison of agencies or regions across the country.

Question: Where can I get information about Hospice Quality Reporting Training?

Answer: Go to www.cms.gov/Medicare/Quality-Initiatives-Patient-Assessment-Instruments/Hospice-Quality-Reporting/Hospice-Quality-Reporting-Training.html for provider training materials and other resources.

CONCLUSION

During the past 15 years, the nature of end-of-life care has been more clearly defined and the dimensions of hospice and palliative care have been identified. Goals of care related to each dimension have been articulated, which has then led to the development of preferred practices and outcomes. Outcome measures have been developed, and monitoring of outcomes is now mandated by Medicare.

References

Dahlin, C. (Ed.). (2013). *Clinical practice guidelines for quality palliative care* (3rd ed.). Pittsburgh, PA: National Consensus Project for Quality Palliative

Care. Retrieved from http://www.nationalconsensusproject.org/NCP_ Clinical_Practice_Guidelines_3rd_Edition.pdf

Dahlin, C. M. (2015). National consensus project for quality palliative care: Promoting excellence in palliative nursing. In B. R. Ferrell, N. Coyle, & J. A. Paice (Eds.), *Oxford textbook of palliative nursing* (pp. 11–19). New York, NY: Oxford University Press.

Institute of Medicine. (2001). *Crossing the quality chasm: A new health system for the 21st century.* Washington, DC: National Academy Press. Retrieved from http://books.nap.edu/openbook.php?record_id=10027

Merriman, M. P. (2011). Measuring outcomes and quality of life. In B. M. Kinzbrunner & J. S. Policzer (Eds.), *End-of-life care: A practical guide* (pp. 103–119). New York, NY: McGraw-Hill.

National Quality Forum. (2006). A national framework and preferred practices for palliative and hospice care quality: A consensus report. Retrieved from http://www.qualityforum.org/publications/2006/12/A_National_ Framework_and_Preferred_Practices_for_Palliative_and_Hospice_ Care_Quality.aspx

National Quality Forum. (2012). NQF endorses palliative and end-of-life care measures. Retrieved from http://www.qualityforum.org/News_And_ Resources/Press_Releases/2012/NQF_Endorses_Palliative_and_End-of -Life_Care_Measures.aspx

15

Monitoring Quality

Today, third-party payers have a vested interest in ensuring that the care they pay for is of the highest quality. Numerous initiatives have been launched to define how quality is measured in end-of-life care settings. The initiatives and the quality measures they spawned are discussed in this chapter.

After reading this chapter, you will be able to:

- Define required reporting structures for hospice
- Discuss the development of a quality assessment and performance improvement (QAPI) plan
- Identify key features of Hospice Item Set (HIS) that must be collected

Fast Facts in a Nutshell

Quality Improvement Organizations (QIOs) work under the direction of the Centers for Medicare & Medicaid Services (CMS) to help ensure that Medicare and Medicaid recipients receive high-quality, consistent care. To identify QIOs in each state, go to www.qualitynet.org, click the "Quality Improvement" tab, then "QIO Directories," then "Quality Innovation Network."

REPORTING REQUIREMENTS

Beginning in 2009, all Medicare-certified hospice programs were required to develop a QAPI plan as part of its Hospice Quality Reporting Program (HQRP) in order to remain eligible for Medicare funding. Specific measures were not required and each hospice developed a QAPI plan that met the unique needs of the organization (National Hospice and Palliative Care Organization, 2009).

However, hospice regulations began to change when the Patient Protection and Affordable Care Act (ACA) was passed in 2010. The regulations included new provisions for quality reporting, but the requirements did not take effect for a few years (fiscal year 2014), allowing time for organizations to align their QAPI plans with the new requirements. For Fiscal Year 2014, hospices were required to submit two quality measures that were set forth by the CMS (2011) as a condition of participation (CoP). These measures were as follows:

- The National Quality Forum (NQF)-endorsed measure related to pain management: Specifically, hospices were required to report the percentage of patients who expressed pain on admission and the percentage of patients who reported that their pain was brought to an acceptable level within 48 hours.
- A structural measure not endorsed by NQF: A hospice organization was required to choose three quality indicators related to patient care such as symptom management, patient safety, or documentation of patient and family goals.

Fast Facts in a Nutshell

According to the CMS (2015), the penalty for failing to submit the required data is a 2% point reduction to the market basket percentage increase for that fiscal year.

Within a few years, the second structural measure, which allowed hospice agencies to choose the aspects of patient care that would be measured, was replaced with a specific set of patient care indicators. The HIS was developed to ensure that all hospices would collect and submit the same data regardless of the patient population or location of the hospice. This approach allows for comparison between and among hospice agencies. HIS can be used to determine compliance with the six measures that were endorsed by the NQF and the one measure that is a modified NQF measure:

- Pain screening
- Pain assessment
- Patients treated with an opioid who are given a bowel regimen
- Dyspnea screening
- Dyspnea treatment
- Treatment preferences
- Beliefs/values addressed

The data collected for the HIS are not direct patient assessment measures. Rather, the data are abstracted via chart review. Thus, documentation in the areas that are included is especially critical for demonstrating that quality care is consistently provided.

Question: Where can I find more information about hospice reporting requirements and CoPs?

Answer: Go to www.federalregister.gov and type "hospice" in the search box. Click on the most recent version of Hospice Wage Index and Payment Rate Update and Hospice Quality Reporting Requirements.

THE HOSPICE CONSUMER ASSESSMENT OF HEALTHCARE PROVIDERS AND SYSTEMS (CAHPS)

In addition to collecting HIS data, as of 2015, it is also mandatory for Medicare-certified hospices to contract with third-party vendors to purchase the CAHPS survey. For 2 years, data will be collected by the vendors and stored in the Hospice CAHPS Data Warehouse. After this period, beginning in Fiscal Year 2018, the vendor will administer the survey and report the results directly to CMS. It is likely that, beginning in 2018, the data will be publicly available. With the implementation of the CAHPS, the Family Evaluation of Hospice Care (FEHC) will no longer be used (Deyta Analytics, 2015).

Fast Facts in a Nutshell

Benchmarking is a process of "comparative evaluation of standard-ization of performance" (Ettorchi-Tardy, Levif, & Michel, 2012, p. e106).

INTERNAL DATA COLLECTION AND QUALITY ASSURANCE

In addition to collecting data on the measures that are required by third-party payers, organizations often wish to choose indicators that are important for helping to monitor the effectiveness of internal protocols and policies. For that purpose, indicators should be chosen that reflect areas important to the organization, its employees, and its patients and families.

The data related to the indicators chosen by Medicare and endorsed by the NQF for the purpose of comparing the quality of care among and between hospices may not be as useful for internal quality monitoring (Dy et al., 2015). Organizations may wish to choose additional indicators that are clinically relevant and could drive internal benchmarking.

Dy et al. (2015) undertook the Measuring What Matters (MWM) project with the goal of identifying internal measures useful in hospice and palliative care settings. After vetting an initial set of 75 indicators, they found 10 indicators that were highly clinically relevant:

- Comprehensive assessment
- Screening for physical symptoms
- Pain treatment
- Dyspnea screening and management
- Discussion of emotional or psychological needs
- Discussion of spiritual or religious concerns
- Documentation of surrogate
- Treatment preferences
- Care consistency with documented care preferences
- A global measure of patient/family perceptions of care

Dy et al. (2015) suggested that specific tools could be used to measure these indicators through chart audits.

CONCLUSION

Reporting requirements for hospices include both internal and external measures. Specific quality indicators include patient-specific components such as pain and symptom management as well as data regarding how well patients' families are supported throughout the hospice experience. Consistent quality monitoring is essential for ensuring quality care within individual hospice agencies and across the country.

References

Centers for Medicare & Medicaid Services. (2011). Hospice wage index for Fiscal Year 2012: Final rule. Retrieved from https://www.gpo.gov/fdsys/pkg/FR-2011-08-04/pdf/2011-19488.pdf

Centers for Medicare & Medicaid Services. (2015). Hospice payment system. Retrieved from https://www.cms.gov/Outreach-and-Education/Medicare-Learning-Network-MLN/MLNProducts/downloads/hospice_pay_sys_fs.pdf

Deyta Analytics. (2015). Hospice CAHPS frequently asked questions. Retrieved from http://www.deyta.com/education-resources/hospice-cahps-frequently-asked-questions

Dy, S. M., Kiley, K. B., Ast, K., Lupu, D., Norton, S. A., McMillan, S. C., . . . & Casarett, D. J. (2015). Measuring what matters: Top-ranked quality indicators for hospice and palliative care from the American Academy of Hospice and Palliative Medicine and Hospice and Palliative Nurses Association. *Journal of Pain and Symptom Management*, 49(4), 773–781. doi:10.1016/j.jpainsymman.2015.01.012

Ettorchi-Tardy, A., Levif, M., & Michel, P. (2012). Benchmarking: A method for continuous quality improvement in health. *Healthcare Policy*, 7(4), e101–e119. Retrieved from http://www.ncbi.nlm.nih.gov/pmc/articles/PMC3359088

National Hospice and Palliative Care Organization. (2009). Hospice QAPI Part I: The QAPI condition of participation. Retrieved from http://www.nhpco.org/sites/default/files/public/regulatory/CMS_QAPI-pt1_%20webcast%20summary.pdf

16

Ensuring Compliance With Hospice Regulations

Today's health care arena is highly regulated and ever-changing. Remaining abreast of the rapid changes in regulations and reporting requirements can be daunting. The purpose of this chapter is to provide an overview of hospice regulations for hospices and to offer resources where the most current information can be found.

After reading this chapter, you will be able to:

- Discuss key points of Medicare regulations for hospices
- Describe quality indicators for hospice and palliative care
- Identify key requirements for changing the patient's level of care

REGULATIONS

The Social Security Act, Section 1861(dd), ensures that hospice care is available and will be covered for Medicare beneficiaries who choose to receive such care from a Medicare-participating hospice (National Hospice and Palliative Care Organization, 2016b). Since most (87.2%) hospice patients are Medicare beneficiaries (National Hospice and Palliative Care Organization, 2014), compliance with Medicare regulations is critical to the success of every hospice organization.

The Secretary of the Department of Health and Human Services (HHS) is responsible for the development of the conditions of participation (CoPs) that a hospice must meet in order to be reimbursed by Medicare or Medicaid for the care provided (National Hospice and Palliative Care Organization, 2016b). The CoPs are outlined, with extensive explanations of the associated requirements, in 42 CFR 418 in the Federal Register and contain information regarding the following hospice-related topics:

- The scope of hospice services
- Patients' rights
- Initial and comprehensive assessment of the patient
- Quality assessment and performance improvement
- Infection control
- Licensed professional services
- Core services (includes bereavement and counseling services)
- Nursing service waiver of requirements that substantially all nursing services be routinely provided directly by a hospice
- Furnishing noncore services
- Physical therapy, occupational therapy, and speech–language pathology
- Waiver of requirement—physical therapy, occupational therapy, speech–language pathology, and dietary counseling
- Hospice aide and homemaker services
- Volunteers
- Organization and administration of services
- Medical director
- Clinical records
- Drugs, biologicals, medical supplies, and durable medical equipment
- Short-term inpatient care
- Hospices that provide inpatient care directly
- Hospices that provide care to residents of a skilled nursing facility, or other residential facility
- Personnel qualifications

The CoPs are enforced to ensure that hospice patients are consistently receiving safe, quality care. State survey agencies conduct surveys of hospices to determine compliance with CoPs. In some cases, approved accreditation agencies may serve as a substitute for state survey agencies. If a hospice is found to not be in compliance with all or some of the CoPs, there can be financial penalties. Ultimately, an agency that does not bring practices into compliance can lose Medicare approval and become ineligible for Medicare/Medicaid funds.

Because of the potential for severe financial repercussions, each hospice agency develops processes to ensure that the CoPs are met. Still, the requirements can be daunting and charting errors or oversights can result in deficiencies. Deficiencies in some areas are more common than in others. Each year, the National Hospice and Palliative Care Organization (2016a) compiles a list of the most common areas of deficiency. A review of this list (see Table 16.1) can help hospice organizations to focus on problem areas.

Fast Facts in a Nutshell

Although there is no limit on the number of days or episodes of general inpatient (GIP) care a patient can receive under the Medicare hospice benefit, this type of inpatient care is intended to be short-term, allowing the patient to return to the home setting once symptoms are managed (National Hospice and Palliative Care Organization, 2012b).

SPECIAL CONDITIONS FOR CHANGE IN LEVEL OF CARE

Hospice was originally intended to allow patients with a terminal illness who choose to forgo curative care to remain at home (routine home care) throughout the trajectory of the disease process with the support of the hospice team members, who manage distressing symptoms and provide support and education for the patient's family. However, patients cannot always remain at home due to the severity of their symptoms and may need more intense medical treatment in an inpatient facility. Also, some patients experience an improvement in their health status, or plateau, and are discharged from hospice service due to a lack of need. A third group of patients includes those who choose to discontinue hospice care in order to seek curative treatments. All three of these groups of patients require special considerations.

Table 16.1

Top Ten Medicare Hospice Recertification Survey Deficiencies

Medicare hospice CoP	Example of the deficiency
1) §418.76: Hospice aide and homemaker services, (h) Standard: Supervision of hospice aides: A registered nurse must make an on-site visit to the patient's home: *No less frequently than every 14 days to assess the quality of care and services provided by the hospice aide and to ensure that services ordered by the hospice interdisciplinary group meet the patient's needs. The hospice aide does not have to be present during this visit.*	Failure to complete or document supervisory visits by RN Failure to complete supervisory visit every 14 days
2) §418.56: Interdisciplinary group, care planning, and coordination of services, (b) Standard: Plan of Care: *All hospice care and services furnished to patients and their families must follow an individualized written plan of care established by the hospice interdisciplinary group in collaboration with the attending physician (if any), the patient or representative, and the primary caregiver in accordance with the patient's needs if any of them so desire. The hospice must ensure that each patient and the primary care giver(s) receive education and training provided by the hospice as appropriate to their responsibilities for the care and services identified in the plan of care.*	Failed to establish, document, or follow plan of care Failure to document assessments of issues noted in the plan of care. For example, if an intervention is part of the plan of care, then nursing assessments should address the ongoing need for the intervention and patient/family teaching regarding the intervention (i.e., oxygen, medications, life chair, etc.)

3) §418.54: Initial and comprehensive assessment of the patient, (c) Standard: Content of the comprehensive assessment, (6): A review of all of the patient's prescription and over-the-counter drugs, herbal remedies and other alternative treatments that could affect drug therapy. This includes, but is not limited to, identification of the following: (i) Effectiveness of drug therapy (ii) Drug side effects (iii) Actual or potential drug interactions (iv) Duplicate drug therapy Drug therapy currently associated with laboratory monitoring.	Failure to add a prescribed medication to the patient's drug profile Duplicate medications included on patient's medication record (e.g., drug listed twice, once with generic name and once with trade name) Failure to list oxygen in medication orders with route, dose, and frequency Failure to document that a recommendation was carried out
4) §418.56: Interdisciplinary group, care planning, and coordination of services, (c) Standard: Content of the plan of care: The hospice must develop an individualized written plan of care for each patient. The plan of care must reflect patient and family goals and interventions based on the problems identified in the initial, comprehensive, and updated comprehensive assessments. The plan of care must include all services necessary for the palliation and management of the terminal illness and related conditions.	Failure to document care specifically required for the individual patient such as wound care, stoma care, ileostomy care, etc. Failure to remove specific items from the plan of care when discontinued such as an IV, Foley catheter, etc. Failure to adjust frequency of interventions, such as dressing changes
5) §418.56: Condition of participation: Interdisciplinary group, care planning, and coordination of services, (c) Standard: Content of the plan of care, (2): A detailed statement of the scope and frequency of services necessary to meet specific patient and family needs.	Failure to document the rationale for services provided and the frequency of visits

(continued)

Table 16.1

Top Ten Medicare Hospice Recertification Survey Deficiencies (continued)

Medicare hospice CoP	Example of the deficiency
6) §418.54: Initial and comprehensive assessment of the patient, (b) Standard: Timeframe for completion of the comprehensive assessment: *The hospice interdisciplinary group, in consultation with the individual's attending physician (if any) must complete the comprehensive assessment no later than 5 calendar days after the election of hospice care in accordance with §418.24.*	Failure to document comprehensive assessment within 5 days of the election of the hospice benefit
7) §418.78: Volunteers, (e) Standard: Level of activity: *Volunteers must provide day-to-day administrative and/or direct patient care services in an amount that, at a minimum, equals 5 percent of the total patient care hours of all paid hospice employees and contract staff. The hospice must maintain records on the use of volunteers for patient care and administrative services, including the type of services and time worked.*	Failure to provide proper training and supervision for volunteers Failure to document the work of volunteers Failure to recruit and assign volunteers for the appropriate number of hours
8) §418.56: Interdisciplinary group, care planning, and coordination of services, (e) Standard: Coordination of services, (2): *Ensure that the care and services are provided in accordance with the plan of care.*	Failure to ensure that all services included in the interdisciplinary plan of care are provided for the patient in a timely manner Failure to document that frequency of visits is consistent with the plan of care

9) §418.56: Interdisciplinary group, care planning, and coordination of services, (d) The hospice interdisciplinary group (in collaboration with the individual's attending physician, if any,) must review, revise, and document the individualized plan as frequently as the patient's condition requires, but no less frequently than every 15 calendar days.

Failure to document that plans of care were reviewed every 14 days by the interdisciplinary team

Failure to update plan of care when the patient's status or family's needs changed

Failure to document team collaboration in the development of the plan of care

10) §418.76: Condition of participation: Hospice aide and homemaker services, (g) Standard: Hospice aide assignments and duties: *Hospice aides are assigned to a specific patient by a registered nurse who is a member of the interdisciplinary group. Written patient care instructions for a hospice aide must be prepared by a registered nurse who is responsible for the supervision of a hospice aide as specified under paragraph (h) of this section.*

Failure to complete supervisory visit or document that it was completed within the required time frame

Failure to document that the care provided by the hospice aide was in accordance with the plan of care

Sources: National Association for Home Care & Hospice (2013); National Hospice and Palliative Care Organization (2012a, 2016a).

Chapter **16** Ensuring Compliance With Hospice Regulations

Inpatient Care

GIP care is defined as a day in which a patient receives care in an inpatient facility for the purpose of managing pain or other symptoms that could not be managed in other settings (National Hospice and Palliative Care Organization, 2012b). It is initiated when:

- Other attempts to manage symptoms have failed.
- A patient experiences a sudden change in condition after a gradual decline.
- Continuous home care has not been effective in alleviating the problem.
- The interdisciplinary team determines that GIP care is the most appropriate level of care.

Supporting documentation is required that outlines:

- The need for GIP care and the circumstances that led to the decision
- What interventions were attempted and the result
- How GIP care will meet the patient's needs (National Hospice and Palliative Care Organization, 2012b)

Other documentation that should be included when GIP care is deemed necessary includes:

- Patient/family involvement and agreement with the change in level of care
- Collaboration between the home care and inpatient staff to ensure a smooth transition of care
- Discharge plans
- A physician's order (National Hospice and Palliative Care Organization, 2012b)

Examples of when GIP care may be appropriate include:

- Pain or symptom crisis that requires frequent assessment and intervention and is not manageable in the current setting
- Intractable nausea and/or vomiting
- Advanced wound care requiring frequent assessment and changes in the treatment plan

- Respiratory distress that is not manageable in the current settings
- Delirium with behavioral issues
- Imminent death—only if there is an associated skilled nursing need

  (National Hospice and Palliative Care Organization, 2012b)

Once it is determined that GIP care is the most appropriate level of care for a particular patient, the patient can be transferred to an inpatient facility that meets Medicare requirements for this type of hospice care. These requirements, according to Standards §418.110 (b) and (e) (Centers for Medicare & Medicaid Services, 2008), specify that an inpatient hospice facility must provide:

- Care in accordance with the patient's plan of care
- Personal care, comfort, and protection from injury, accident, or infection
- An RN on each shift
- A home-like atmosphere that is designed to promote the dignity, comfort, and privacy of the patient
- A private space for family consults, meetings, and visiting
- Physical space for the family after the patient's death
- Open visiting hours with no restrictions on the ages of the visitors

Although many hospice organizations operate an inpatient facility, some do not. Those that do not may contract with other agencies to provide inpatient services. According to the National Hospice and Palliative Care Organization (2012b), when GIP care is provided in a contracted facility:

- The hospice interdisciplinary team is responsible for managing patient care according to the plan of care.
- Visits from the hospice staff must occur to ensure coordination of care, and ongoing communication with the patient and family.
- Daily visits from the hospice staff are recommended.

The proposed fiscal year 2017 hospice payment rates are as follows:

Routine Home Care (days 1–60): $190.41
Routine Home Care (days 60+): $149.68
Continuous Home Care (24 hours): $963.69
Inpatient Respite Care: $170.80
General Inpatient Care: $734.22

Source: Centers for Medicare & Medicare Services (2016).

Throughout the course of the inpatient admission, the goal is to manage the patient's symptoms and successfully transition the patient to routine care. Achieving this goal is made possible through effective discharge planning that begins when the patient is admitted to the inpatient facility and continues throughout the patient's stay. Documentation should include:

- How the patient is responding to interventions in the inpatient setting
- The type and strength of family and community support available to the patient after discharge
- How and when the patient will be discharged
- The level of care that will be required after discharge (National Hospice and Palliative Care Organization, 2012b)

Patient Discharge—Improved Condition

The hospice benefit is extended to patients who have a life expectancy of about 6 months if the disease runs its course without curative intervention. If a patient's condition improves or does not decline during the 6-month period, or if the patient moves out of the service area, the hospice interdisciplinary team may determine that the patient is no longer eligible for hospice services and the hospice "must file a notice of termination/revocation of election (NOTR) with the Medicare contractor within 5 calendar days after the effective date of the discharge or revocation, unless the hospice has already filed a final claim for the beneficiary" (National Hospice and Palliative Care Organization, 2016b, p. 11). According to the National Hospice and

Palliative Care Organization (2016b), when a patient is discharged from hospice:

- A live discharge order must be obtained from the hospice physician
- The attending physician must be consulted prior to discharge, and this should be documented in the health record

Discharge from hospice services has implications for both the patient and the hospice organization. After discharge, the patient:

- Is no longer under the care of the hospice
- May resume Medicare coverage of the benefits that were waived when the patient elected hospice benefits, but may elect hospice care at any time in the future if eligible

The hospice agency must:

- Have a discharge process in place that outlines the process of discharge in cases where the patient's condition improves or stabilizes, or the patient is otherwise ineligible for services
- Provide any necessary family counseling or other necessary services prior to the patient's discharge

Patient Discharge—Revocation of Hospice Benefits

Every hospice patient may revoke his or her election of hospice benefits at any time in writing. On the day that the revocation of benefits is signed by the patient, hospice care ends and the patient is eligible for the Medicare benefits that were waived when the election of hospice benefits was signed. The patient may elect the hospice benefit at any time in the future if eligible for services (National Hospice and Palliative Care Organization, 2016b).

CONCLUSION

This chapter provided an overview of the regulations and CoPs that apply to Medicare-approved hospices, including special circumstances such as patient discharge and transfers to GIP level of care. Common areas of deficiencies were reviewed, and examples of the deficiencies were illustrated. Tips for ensuring compliance were offered.

References

Centers for Medicare & Medicaid Services. (2008). Medicare & Medicaid programs: Hospice conditions of participation. Retrieved from https://www.gpo.gov/fdsys/pkg/FR-2008-06-05/pdf/08-1305.pdf

Centers for Medicare & Medicaid Services. (2016). Medicare program; FY 2017 hospice wage index and payment rate update and hospice quality reporting requirements. Retrieved from https://www.federalregister.gov/articles/2016/04/28/2016-09631/medicare-program-fy-2017-hospice-wage-index-and-payment-rate-update-and-hospice-quality-reporting

National Association for Home Care & Hospice. (2013). Hospice: Top 10 deficiencies. Retrieved from http://www.nahc.org/NAHCReport/nr130408_1

National Hospice and Palliative Care Organization. (2012a). CMS FY 2011 top ten hospice survey deficiencies compliance recommendations. Retrieved from http://www.nhpco.org/sites/default/files/public/regulatory/CMS_TopTenHospiceSurveyDeficiencies.pdf

National Hospice and Palliative Care Organization. (2012b). Managing general inpatient care for symptom management: Tips for providers. Retrieved from http://www.nhpco.org/sites/default/files/public/regulatory/GIP_Tip_GIP_Sheet.pdf

National Hospice and Palliative Care Organization. (2014). NHPCO's facts and figures: Hospice care in America, 2014 Edition. Retrieved from http://www.nhpco.org/sites/default/files/public/Statistics_Research/2014_Facts_Figures.pdf

National Hospice and Palliative Care Organization. (2016a). CMS top ten hospice survey deficiencies comparison. Retrieved from http://www.nhpco.org/sites/default/files/public/regulatory/Survey_deficiency_compare_2013-2015.pdf

National Hospice and Palliative Care Organization. (2016b). Hospice policy compendium: The Medicare hospice benefit, regulations, quality reporting, and public policy. Retrieved from http://www.nhpco.org/sites/default/files/public/public_policy/Hospice_Policy_Compendium.pdf

17

Electronic Documentation in Hospice

Electronic documentation is a tool that helps health care professionals document the care they provide in a succinct and uniform way. Several initiatives have been implemented to encourage the use of electronic documentation in hospice. This chapter discusses general information about electronic charting and documentation tips specific to hospice.

After reading this chapter, you will be able to:

- Discuss the use of electronic charting in hospice
- Identify incentives for the use of electronic health records
- Describe proper hospice documentation

Fast Facts in a Nutshell

"Electronic medical records (EMRs) are increasingly viewed as essential tools for quality assurance and improvement in many care settings" (Zheng, Rokoske, Kirk, Lyda-McDonald, & Bernard, 2014, p. 582).

ELECTRONIC DOCUMENTATION

Most quality reporting is done through medical chart review. Use of electronic records allows easier access to vital information and more uniform documentation. Further, health care providers are more likely to document components of quality if prompted to do so within the electronic health record. Thus, use of electronic records is one way to improve compliance and monitor quality (Cagle et al., 2012). Electronic health records also allow remote access to charts, and improve overall patient care (King, Patel, Jamoom, & Furukawa, 2013). Advantages of electronic charting include:

- Improved access to interdisciplinary notes
- Automatic prompting to document key items
- Uniform documentation by all providers
- Easier access to needed information

Barriers to the use of electronic charting include:

- Implementation costs
- Staff training
- Limited availability of software that is hospice-appropriate
- Lack of system compatibility
  (Cagle et al., 2012)

ELECTRONIC HEALTH RECORD INCENTIVE PROGRAM

The American Recovery and Reinvestment Act of 2009 established incentives for the incorporation of electronic health records. The goal of expanding the adoption of health information technology, such as electronic health records, is to promote continuous quality improvement and information exchange at the point of care. In order to participate in the incentive program, an organization must demonstrate meaningful use of health information technology (Centers for Medicare & Medicaid Services, 2016).

"Meaningful use" means that hospice organizations will use electronic health records to (HealthIT.gov, 2015a):

- Improve the quality of patient care
- Increase collaboration with patients and families

- Promote care coordination
- Improve the privacy and security of health information

The ultimate goals of the incentive program are (HealthIT.gov, 2015a):

- Improving clinical outcomes
- Increasing efficiency
- Empowering patients through easier access to their own medical records

Following are the three stages of the incentive program (Centers for Medicare & Medicaid Services, 2016; HealthIT.gov, 2015a):

- Stage 1 (2011–2012): Data collection and sharing
- Stage 2 (2014): Advanced clinical processes
- Stage 3 (2016): Improved outcomes

To attain meaningful use and receive the incentive payments, hospice organizations must demonstrate that use of the electronic health record has enabled streamlined processes; enhanced communication within the hospice team, with other providers, as well as patients and families; improved patient safety; and improved patient and family access to self-management tools (HealthIT.gov, 2015b). Meaningful use also enables standardized documentation of assessments, interventions, and outcomes, which promotes uniform patient care.

Fast Facts in a Nutshell

Electronic documentation is a useful tool for collecting data related to quality and compliance (Cagle et al., 2012).

DOCUMENTATION TIPS

Patients' medical records are the main source of the information regarding each patient's status and response to interventions. So, nurses' documentation must be complete and accurate, reflecting the excellent interdisciplinary care the patient and family receives. In addition to completing the required sections of the electronic health record as prompted, nurses also complete a narrative section of the chart, which allows the opportunity to "paint the picture" of what the patient and family are experiencing and how their needs are being met. This involves (Cosmos Hospice, LLC, n.d.):

- Thorough documentation of the initial assessment
- Plan of care and problems, interventions, and goals (PIGs)
- Global assessment of the patient's condition
- Focused assessment findings for systems where problems are noted
- Noting level of pain, pain management interventions, and their effectiveness
- Patient and family teaching
- Supervision of hospice aide (every 2 weeks—hospice aide does not need to be present)
- Supervision of LPN/LVN (every month—LPN/LVN must be observed)
- Signs of declining status, including physical, psychosocial, and spiritual needs
- Interventions implemented by all members of the interdisciplinary team to meet the patient's or family's needs

RECERTIFICATION DOCUMENTATION

Documentation related to recertification must be completed on a regular basis. Hospice nurses assess each patient and document the continued need for hospice care. Some ways to ensure that recertification documentation is incorporated into the patient's medical record on an ongoing basis include documentation of (CGS Administrators, LLC, 2013a):

- All services furnished, whether by the hospice or through a contract with another organization
- Progression of the terminal illness and that the patient's life expectancy is 6 months or less
- Objective data to support continuation of hospice services
- Appropriateness of the patient's level of care

When documenting clinical findings during recertification periods, hospice nurses document additional information to support the continuation of hospice services such as:

- Physical changes such as decreased body mass index, mid-arm circumference, or decrease in appetite
- Declining functional status
- Increased psychosocial needs
- Recurrent aspiration or infections
- Signs of decline such as edema, agitation, decreased blood pressure, changes in respiratory pattern, weakness, and decubiti
- Symptoms such as cough, dyspnea, new or persistent pain, seizures, and dysphagia
- Altered lab results (only if available)
- Changes in Karnofsky Performance Scale (KPS)/Palliative Performance Scale (PPS) scores, Functional Assessment Staging Test (FAST) score (for patients with dementia only), or Eastern Cooperative Oncology Group (ECOG) score
- New medications required to manage symptoms (CGS Administrators, LLC, 2013b)

CONCLUSION

Documentation in every nursing specialty, including hospice, should include a thorough assessment of the patient's condition and responses to interventions. Hospice documentation should also address findings that support ongoing hospice services for the patient's terminal condition. In this chapter, general documentation tips were reviewed that help ensure the collection of data required for quality monitoring as well as information that specifically supports terminality and the need for hospice care.

References

Cagle, J. G., Rokoske, F. S., Durham, D., Schenk, A. P., Spence, C., & Hanson, L. C. (2012). Use of electronic documentation for quality improvement in hospice. *American Journal of Medical Quality, 27*(4), 282–290. doi:10.1177/1062860611425103

Centers for Medicare & Medicaid Services. (2016). Electronic health records (EHR) incentive programs. Retrieved from https://www.cms.gov/Regulations-and-Guidance/Legislation/EHRIncentivePrograms/index.html?redirect=/ehrincentiveprograms

CGS Administrators, LLC. (2013a). Hospice documentation. Retrieved from http://www.cgsmedicare.com/hhh/coverage/coverage_guidelines/hospice_documentation.html

CGS Administrators, LLC. (2013b). Appropriate clinical factors to consider during recertification of Medicare hospice patients. Retrieved from https://www.cgsmedicare.com/hhh/education/materials/pdf/hospice_clinical_factors_recert_tool_h-020-01_07-2011.pdf

Cosmos Hospice, LLC. (n.d.). Nursing documentation: Paint the picture. Retrieved from http://www.joshlangfielddesigns.com/sites/cosmoshospice.com/custom/pdf/PAINT_THE_PICTURE.pdf

HealthIT.gov. (2015a). Meaningful use: Definition and objectives. Retrieved from https://www.healthit.gov/providers-professionals/meaningful-use-definition-objectives

HealthIT.gov. (2015b). How to attain meaningful use. Retrieved from https://www.healthit.gov/providers-professionals/how-attain-meaningful-use

King, J., Patel, V., Jamoom, E. W., & Furukawa, M. F. (2013). Clinical benefits of electronic health record use: National findings. *Health Services Research*, *49*(1), 391–404. doi:10.1111/1475-6773.12135

Zheng, N. T., Rokoske, F. S., Kirk, M. A., Lyda-McDonald, B., & Bernard, S. L. (2014). Hospices' use of electronic medical records for quality assessment and performance improvement programs. *Journal of Pain and Symptom Management*, *48*(4), 582–589. doi:10.1016/j.jpainsymman.2013.11.010

V

Occupational Stress in Hospice Nursing

18

Sources of Occupational Stress

A career in nursing is inherently fraught with numerous stressors. Nurses are on the front line of human suffering on a daily basis. Yet, they are expected to be at their best at all times. Hospice nurses, specifically, work with patients who are preparing for their own deaths and families who are working toward letting go of someone dear to them. In these difficult circumstances, hospice nurses are expected to simultaneously provide support for patients and families, control their own emotions, and work through the losses of multiple patients. Other job-related stressors, such as office politics and interpersonal conflict, can also add a significant burden. This chapter addresses the sources of stress for nurses.

After reading this chapter, you will be able to:

- Identify sources of occupational stress for hospice nurses
- Describe workplace factors that increase occupational stress
- Discuss the effects of personality types and generational differences in the workplace

OCCUPATIONAL STRESS AND HOSPICE NURSING

Occupational stress, also called "job stress," is defined as a harmful physical and emotional response that occurs when the requirements of a job are mismatched to the abilities of the workers, the resources provided by the employer, or the expectations of the employer (Najimi,

Goudarzi, & Sharifirad, 2012; Roberts, Grubb, & Grosch, 2012). Occupational stress can also be related to dynamics such as workload and the nature of the job (Orly, Rivka, Rivka, & Dorit, 2012). Each day, hospice nurses face stressors in the office, on the road, in patients' homes, and while on call. Hospice nurses who work in inpatient settings face similar stressors during their shifts. Some sources of occupational stress for nurses include (Happell et al., 2013; Roberts et al., 2012):

- Heavy workloads
- Unsupportive management
- Shift work and long work hours
- On-call requirements
- Handover procedures
- Lack of professional progression/opportunity
- Lack of control
- Interpersonal conflict
- Bullying and physical violence
- Insufficient resources
- Poor reward systems

Fast Facts in a Nutshell

According to the World Health Organization (2016 , para. 1), a healthy job is "likely to be one where the pressures on employees are appropriate in relation to their abilities and resources, to the amount of control they have over their work, and to the support they receive from people who matter to them."

Stressors specific to hospice nursing include (Peters et al., 2012; Tunnah, Johnstone, & Jones, 2012):

- Frequent exposure to death and dying
- Family grieving
- Family conflict
- High workloads
- Workload pressure
- Lack of a support system/isolation
- Psychological distress related to frequently facing existential issues

- Communication issues with the interdisciplinary team
- Inadequate preparation for providing end-of-life care

LATERAL VIOLENCE AND WORKPLACE BULLYING

One serious issue that has been repeatedly identified as a source of occupational stress for nurses is lateral violence, which is sometimes called "workplace bullying." Lateral violence is defined as behavior that consistently causes an individual or group to feel belittled, degraded, intimidated, or harassed in the workplace. Workplace bullying can also include exclusion of certain individuals or groups (Allen, Holland, & Reynolds, 2015).

Fast Facts in a Nutshell

Nurse–nurse bullying undermines patient care and reduces the work performance of nurses (Hutchinson & Jackson, 2013).

Aggression in the workplace may manifest in any number of ways, including blatant disregard for mutual respect within the workplace or low-level incivilities such as ignoring or excluding coworkers from activities (Taylor & Kluemper, 2012). Workplace bullies undermine and demean their coworkers and rally the support of others against the target to reinforce aggressive behaviors and further isolate the target (Becher & Visovsky, 2012). Some examples of aggressive behaviors in the workplace include:

- Criticizing
- Intimidation
- Blaming
- Fighting
- Refusing to help
- Public humiliation
- Withholding behaviors (silent treatment, exclusion, or omission)
- Name calling
- Threatening behaviors or actions
- Gossiping
- Isolating

- Ignoring
- Giving unreasonable assignments
  (Becher & Visovsky, 2012)

Lateral violence, also called "horizontal violence," is especially prevalent in nursing, with more than half (61%) of nurses reporting that they experienced horizontal violence in the workplace (Becher & Visovsky, 2012). Lateral violence results in psychological and physical issues such as:

- Headaches
- Stress
- Impatience
- Nervousness
- Impaired sleep
- Diminished social skills
- Depression
- Inability to concentrate
- Inability to cope with stressors
- Posttraumatic stress disorder
  (Allen et al., 2015)

Other factors also contribute to stress in the work environment. For example, the way that personalities blend or clash within the team can have a profound effect on occupational stress.

PERSONALITY TYPES IN THE WORKPLACE

Several ways to categorize personalities have been developed. One of the first personality trait models, the "Big Five Trait Taxonomy," has been studied extensively (John, Naumann, & Soto, 2008). The model includes five main personality types and descriptors of each type, which are summarized in Table 18.1.

Question: Where can I find more information on occupational health initiatives?
Answer: See the National Institute for Occupational Safety and Health's website at www.cdc.gov/niosh.

Table 18.1

Personality Types	
Type	**Descriptors**
Extraversion	Talkative, assertive, energetic, active, outgoing, outspoken, dominant, forceful, enthusiastic, sociable
Agreeableness	Sympathetic, kind, appreciative, affectionate, soft-hearted, warm, generous, trusting, helpful
Conscientiousness	Organized, thorough, efficient, reliable, conscientious, precise, practical, deliberate, cautious
Neuroticism	Tense, anxious, nervous, moody, worrying, touchy, high-strung, dependent, emotional
Openness	Wide interests, imaginative, intelligent, original, insightful, curious, artistic, clever, inventive

Source: John et al. (2008).

Some organizations use personality trait tests, such as the Myers-Briggs Type Indicator® (MBTI), to help employees identify the way their own personality traits influence their work styles and preferences. Sometimes, employees are invited to share the results of the inventory as a team-building exercise.

Those who take the inventory identify whether they are more extroverted or introverted, rely more on sensing or intuition, approach decision making through thinking or feeling, and whether they are more judging or perceiving. These traits are also thought to influence one's penchant for gathering data and making final and binding decisions or whether one prefers to engage in ongoing consideration of further data and make more fluid plans with the intention of making adjustments as new information becomes available (The Myers & Briggs Foundation, 2016).

GENERATIONAL DIFFERENCES IN THE WORKPLACE

Generational differences factor into how a work team functions. Putre (2013) noted that three main generations are found in today's workplace:

- Baby boomers (born between 1946 and 1964)
- Generation X (born between 1965 and 1985)
- Generation Y, or Millennials (born between 1985 and 2000)

Fast Facts in a Nutshell

Work values vary due to generational differences, and this can cause friction. Knowledge of these differences can foster changes that make the workplace better for all employees (Gursoy, Chi, & Karadag, 2013).

Generations are thought to share certain characteristics and worldviews, which contribute to their workflow preferences and job attitudes. When employees who are part of one generation expect all of their coworkers to share their views, friction can occur. In general, generations differ in terms of their:

- Personalities
- Work values
- Attitudes toward work
- Leadership and teamwork preferences
- Leader behaviors
- Career expectations
  (Lyons & Kuron, 2014)

In health care settings, these differences can manifest in workers' shift preferences, assignment preferences, and how they respond to leadership and management styles. Putre (2013) and Acar (2014) generalized work preferences according to generations in the following way:

- *Baby boomers* expect recognition for their loyalty and dedication to the organization. They prefer face-to-face communication to electronic communication. Baby boomers are rule-bound and seek clear lines of authority. They are willing to come to work on short notice and to sacrifice personal time for the demands of their jobs.
- Members of *Generation X* are more self-reliant than baby boomers and are interested in developing a transferrable skill set. They prefer a good work–life balance. They value mobility and will change jobs to gain the balance and work environment they want. Gen Xers are very adaptable to new technology and seek new challenges in the workplace. They respond well to positive feedback and seek rationale for changes in assignments or new rules.

- Members of *Generation Y* seek jobs that they can integrate with their personal lives. They do not prioritize their jobs over family and/or friends, and are willing to change jobs readily. Gen Yers are excellent multitaskers and are frequently in touch with others through electronic means and social media. They tend to be more informal with peers than previous generations. At work, they seek rewards for their efforts and expect reasonable rationale for the rules.

Friction in the workplace can emerge from a lack of understanding of a coworker's perspective and needs. Also, generational differences can develop when a member of one generation feels slighted or judged. Members of Generations X and Y share more common ground with each other than with the baby boomers, but their viewpoints still differ in the areas of teamwork, with Gen Xers being more individualistic (Acar, 2014). Some ways to alleviate generational friction in the workplace are to (Kennedy, 2003; Putre, 2013):

- Encourage workers to prioritize what is important to them
- Recognize the hard work and dedication of all employees
- Develop learning activities that allow older and younger workers to learn from each other
- Encourage longevity by providing positive feedback, opportunities for advancement, and time for employees to gather informally at activities such as awards or holiday events
- Design team-building exercises that encourage members of different generations to rely on and trust each other

CONCLUSION

For nurses, sources of stress include the nature of the work, job expectations, lack of support from management, and general workplace differences among workers such as personality types and generational styles. These factors can diminish employees' devotion to their work and the mission of the organization and result in serious consequences for both the individual workers and the organization as a whole.

References

Acar, A. B. (2014). Do intrinsic and extrinsic motivation factors differ for Generation X and Generation Y? *International Journal of Business and Social Science*, 5(5), 12–20. Retrieved from http://www.ijbssnet.com

Allen, B. C., Holland, P., & Reynolds, R. (2015). The effect of bullying on burnout in nurses: The moderating role of psychological detachment. *Journal of Advanced Nursing, 71*(2), 381–390. doi:10.1111/jan.12489

Becher, J., & Visovsky, C. (2012). Horizontal violence in nursing. *Medsurg Nursing, 21*(4), 210–213. Retrieved from https://amsn.org/professional-development/periodicals/medsurg-nursing-journal

Gursoy, D., Chi, C.-G. Q., & Karadag, E. (2013). Generational differences in work values and attitudes among frontline and service contact employees. *International Journal of Hospitality Management, 32*, 40–48. doi:10.1016/j.ijhm.2012.04.002

Happell, B., Dwyer, T., Reid-Searl, K., Burke, K. J., Caperchione, C. M., & Gaskin, C. J. (2013). Nurses and stress: Recognizing causes and seeking solutions. *Journal of Nursing Management, 21*(4), 638–647. doi:10.1111/jonm.12037

Hutchinson, M., & Jackson, D. (2013). Hostile clinician behaviours in the nursing work environment and implications for patient care: A mixed-methods systematic review. *BMC Nursing, 12*(1), 25. Retrieved from https://bmcnurs.biomedcentral.com

John, O. P., Naumann, L. P., & Soto, C. J. (2008). Paradigm shift to the integrative big five trait taxonomy: History, measurement, and conceptual issues. In O. P. John, R. W. Robins, & L. A. Pervin (Eds.), *Handbook of personality: Theory and research* (3rd ed., pp. 114–155). New York, NY: Guilford Press.

Kennedy, M. M. (2003). Managing different generations requires new skills, insightful leadership. *Physician Executive, 29*(6), 20–24. Retrieved from http://acpe.physicianleaders.org/publications/pej

Lyons, S., & Kuron, L. (2014). Generational differences in the workplace: A review of the evidence and directions for future research. *Journal of Organizational Behavior, 35*(S1), S139–S157. Retrieved from http://onlinelibrary.wiley.com/journal/10.1002/(ISSN)1099-1379

The Myers & Briggs Foundation. (2016). MBTI® basics. Retrieved from http://www.myersbriggs.org/my-mbti-personality-type/mbti-basics

Najimi, A., Goudarzi, A. M., & Sharifirad, G. (2012). Causes of job stress in nurses: A cross-sectional study. *Iranian Journal of Nursing and Midwifery Research, 17*(4), 301–305. Retrieved from http://www.ncbi.nlm.nih.gov/pmc/articles/PMC3702151

Orly, S., Rivka, B., Rivka, E., & Dorit, S. E. (2012). Are cognitive–behavioral interventions effective in reducing occupational stress among nurses? *Applied Nursing Research, 25*(3), 152–157. doi:10.1016/j.apnr.2011.01.004

Peters, L., Cant, R., Sellick, K., O'Connor, M., Lee, S., Burney, S., & Karimi, L. (2012). Is work stress in palliative care nurses a cause for concern? A literature review. *International Journal of Palliative Nursing, 18*(11), 561–567. Retrieved from http://www.magonlinelibrary.com/toc/ijpn/18/11

Putre, L. (2013, January). Generations in the workplace. *Hospitals & Health Networks.* Retrieved from www.hhnmag.com

Roberts, R., Grubb, P. L., & Grosch, J. W. (2012, June 25). Alleviating job stress in nurses. *Medscape*. Retrieved from www.medscape.com

Taylor, S. G., & Kluemper, D. H. (2012). Linking perceptions of role stress and incivility to workplace aggression: The moderating role of personality. *Journal of Occupational Health Psychology*, *17*(3), 316–329. doi:10.1037/a0028211

Tunnah, K., Johnstone, R., & Jones, A. (2012). Stress in hospice at home nurses: A qualitative study. *BMJ Supportive & Palliative Care*, *2*(Suppl. 1), A26. Retrieved from http://spcare.bmj.com

World Health Organization. (2016). Occupational health: Stress at the workplace. Retrieved from http://www.who.int/occupational_health/topics/stressatwp/en

19

Consequences of Occupational Stress

Chronic occupational stress is detrimental to the health and well-being of employees. It has both psychological and physical effects that can lead to consequences not only for the individual but also for the employer. Stress-related health issues interfere with productivity, decrease retention, and drive up the costs of health plans for employers. This chapter reviews the consequences of occupational stress on both employees and employers, with an emphasis on the cyclical nature of their relationship.

After reading this chapter, you will be able to:

- Identify consequences of occupational stress for employees
- Identify consequences of occupational stress for organizations
- Describe the cycle of occupational stress

CONSEQUENCES OF OCCUPATIONAL STRESS ON EMPLOYEES

Effects of chronic stress in the workplace can lead to (Ekundayo, 2014; Roberts, Grubb, & Grosch, 2012):

- Increased absenteeism
- Disengagement
- Diminished job satisfaction

- Decreased productivity
- Work-related injuries
- Low morale
- Burnout
- Compassion fatigue
- Psychological distress including anxiety, depression, fatigue, and low self-esteem
- Physical consequences such as hypertension, ulcers, migraines, and immunosuppression

Several of these factors have been explored extensively in relation to the nursing profession. Specifically, burnout and compassion fatigue are consequences of the work-related stressors that nurses face regularly.

Fast Facts in a Nutshell

Nurses who find meaning in their work are less likely to experience burnout (Rosales, Labrague, & Rosales, 2013).

EFFECTS OF CHRONIC STRESS ON NURSES: BURNOUT AND COMPASSION FATIGUE

Compared with other health care providers, nurses are more prone to burnout (Rosales et al., 2013). Burnout results from chronic workplace stress and is characterized by physical, emotional, and psychological exhaustion (Allen, Holland, & Reynolds, 2015). Signs of burnout include (Bisk, 2016):

- Constant fatigue
- Feeling overworked
- Feeling underappreciated
- Lack of enthusiasm about work
- Compassion fatigue

Compassion fatigue plagues those whose work involves communicating compassion for those who need emotional support. Compassion fatigue develops over time as a result of chronic work stress. Compassion fatigue involves (Hegney et al., 2014):

- Behavioral changes
- Inability to demonstrate compassion for patients and families
- Sadness
- Depression
- Anxiety
- Intrusive thoughts
- Flashbacks
- Emotional numbness
- Avoidance
- Cynicism
- Poor self-esteem
- Survivor guilt

Fast Facts in a Nutshell

An employee can pinpoint the cause of *acute stress*. When the stressor is removed, the individual's performance returns to normal. *Chronic stress* results from unrelenting pressure that has no foreseeable end. The employee feels professionally exhausted and may become disengaged from the workplace (Ekundayo, 2014).

Nurses who experience burnout and compassion fatigue are less able to provide the type of care that they would ideally like to provide. This leads to poor professional self-image and decreased job satisfaction. When nurses are not satisfied with their jobs, quality of patient care suffers (Rosales et al., 2013), which has a negative effect on nurses, patients, and organizations.

THE EFFECTS OF EMPLOYEE STRESS ON ORGANIZATIONS

When employees are chronically stressed and cannot contribute to their full potential, productivity decreases. Disengaged employees manifest the following behaviors, which can spread throughout the workplace (Ekundayo, 2014):

- Decreased performance
- Decreased motivation
- Decreased commitment

- Increased dissatisfaction
- Increased absenteeism
- Increased formal grievances
- Increased turnover

Disengaged workers and lack of productivity derail the mission and goals of an organization. Therefore, it is in the best interests of the organization and the individual employee to address sources of occupational stress because as stress increases, productivity decreases (Orly, Rivka, Rivka, & Dorit, 2012). As worker productivity decreases, the organizational system is stressed. This dynamic causes employers to pressure employees, which, in turn, causes additional employee stress. This cycle is depicted in Figure 19.1.

Decreased commitment, lack of job satisfaction, and lack of commitment to the mission of the organization can prompt employees to seek employment elsewhere. Although employers may feel that employee attrition, particularly attrition of unmotivated workers, can help

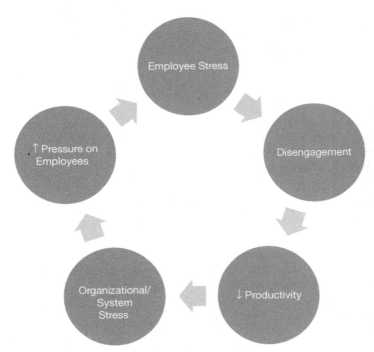

Figure 19.1 Cycle of occupational stress.

strengthen an organization, high turnover is financially costly and damaging to teams. The cost of workplace stress is estimated to be $300 billion annually, which includes the cost of employee turnover, absenteeism, and low productivity (Taylor & Kluemper, 2012).

CONCLUSION

Given the serious consequences of occupational stress, it is in the best interests of employers and employees to partner in order to develop programs and skills that minimize job stress. Interventions aimed at breaking the cycle of occupational stress could help improve workplace harmony.

References

Allen, B. C., Holland, P., & Reynolds, R. (2015). The effect of bullying on burnout in nurses: The moderating role of psychological detachment. *Journal of Advanced Nursing, 71*(2), 381–390. doi:10.1111/jan.12489

Ekundayo, J. A. (2014). Occupational stress and employees' productivity in the workplace. *International Journal of Scientific Research in Education, 7*(2), 157–165. Retrieved from http://www.ijsre.com/index.html

Hegney, D. G., Craigie, M., Hemsworth, D., Osseiran-Moisson, R., Francis, K., & Drury, V. (2014). Compassion satisfaction, compassion fatigue, anxiety, depression and stress in registered nurses in Australia: Study 1 results. *Journal of Nursing Management, 22*(4), 506–518. doi:10.1111/jonm.12160

Orly, S., Rivka, B., Rivka, E., & Dorit, S.-E. (2012). Are cognitive–behavioral interventions effective in reducing occupational stress among nurses? *Applied Nursing Research, 25*(3), 152–157. doi:10.1016/j.apnr.2011.01.004

Roberts, R., Grubb, P. L., & Grosch, J. W. (2012, June 25). Alleviating job stress in nurses. *Medscape.* Retrieved from www.medscape.com

Rosales, R. A., Labrague, L. J., & Rosales, G. L. (2013). Nurses' job satisfaction and burnout: Is there a connection? *International Journal of Advanced Nursing Studies, 2*(1), 1–10. Retrieved from http://www.sciencepubco.com/index.php/IJANS

Taylor, S. G., & Kluemper, D. H. (2012). Linking perceptions of role stress and incivility to workplace aggression: The moderating role of personality. *Journal of Occupational Health Psychology, 17*(3), 316–329. doi:10.1037/a0028211

University of South Florida Health. (2016). Signs you're experiencing nurse burnout. Retrieved from http://www.usfhealthonline.com/resources/career/signs-you-are-experiencing-nurse-burnout/#.V5LVL_krJD9

20

Addressing Occupational Stress

Both employees and employers suffer the consequences of workplace stress. Several strategies can be used to minimize occupational stress and decrease interpersonal conflict and toxicity in the workplace.

After reading this chapter, you will be able to:

- Identify approaches to mitigating workplace stress
- Navigate a toxic workplace
- Identify the steps of conflict resolution

STRATEGIES TO MINIMIZE OCCUPATIONAL STRESS

Employers have traditionally used two different approaches to address workplace stress. The first is to address organization culture and processes. To do this, management focuses on (Orly, Rivka, Rivka, & Dorit, 2012; Roberts, Grubb, & Grosch, 2012):

- Internal processes
- Management practices
- Workflow issues
- Employee assignments/workload
- Clearly defining employee expectations

- Improving communication
- Providing opportunities for positive social interactions among employees
- Reducing uncertainty about career ladders

Individual managers can help alleviate occupational stress by:

- Regularly recognizing employees' contributions
- Monitoring assignments to be sure they are manageable
- Listening to employees and making changes as needed to improve working conditions
- Monitoring internal stress and taking steps to manage it
- Recognizing that change is a challenge for employees and offering support through times of transition
- Making small gestures, such as leaving a card signed by office mates on employees' birthdays or work anniversaries, to show employees they matter
- Offering to pitch in and help when workers are overwhelmed

Another approach to reducing occupational stress is to focus on employees through targeted educational or stress-reduction programs. For example, employers might offer:

- Meditation areas
- Exercise programs
- Wellness programs, including weight management and addictions counseling
- Cognitive behavioral therapies
- Stress-reduction skill-building sessions, such as time management programs
- In-services on conflict resolution
- Team-building activities

Workplaces bring together individuals from varied backgrounds and levels of professional experience in one setting. Ideally, all the talents of a diverse team would be brought to bear within an organization, maximizing productivity. However, individual personalities, workflow preferences, and problem-solving approaches can vary so greatly that a team can devolve into conflict when faced with stressful situations.

CONFLICT RESOLUTION

Conflict occurs when two or more people disagree and is almost inevitable in work situations where many personalities and work styles come together (Dahlin & Wittenberg, 2015; Tjosvold, Wong, & Yi Feng Chen, 2014). Mallidi (2015) noted that engaging in successful conflict resolution helps build leadership skills. But, before one can take on the task of resolving conflict, it is important to recognize the various ways individuals handle conflict. The four main styles are as follows (Saltman, 2006, as cited by Mallidi, 2015):

- **Avoidance:** In this approach, the person simply sidesteps the issue, which may be appropriate when the issue is not significant. However, it is not effective when the issue is ongoing or significant.
- **Accommodation:** With this approach, the person listens carefully to the other person and accepts his or her position. This is a good approach when a person understands that his or her own position is flawed.
- **Competition:** With this approach, the person forcefully defends his or her own position. The approach does not support good teamwork.
- **Collaboration:** Using this approach, each person involved in the conflict engages in negotiation to find a solution that meets everyone's needs. This is generally considered the most effective style of resolving conflict.

The approaches to conflict resolution tend to vary according to a person's personal preference, as well as the perceived power differential in a given situation. When conflict occurs, the steps of navigating a resolution are as follows (Dahlin & Wittenberg, 2015):

- Gathering facts about the conflict
- Identifying the goal of conflict resolution
- Addressing the conflict with the other person or persons involved
- Identifying each person's stake in resolving the conflict
- Discussing the conflict
- Engaging in problem solving
- Determining outcomes that meet the needs of both parties

When conflict is resolved successfully, it can be a constructive process that results in mutual benefit (Tjosvold et al., 2014). However, when conflict is very challenging or deep-rooted and ongoing, mediation may be beneficial.

MEDIATION

Mediation is a process in which conflict is resolved through a third party whose interest is in encouraging reflection and enhancing communication among parties. Typically, the need for mediation arises from disputes about budgets, staffing, or direction within a workplace. The purpose of mediation is primarily to rebuild relationships (Brubaker, Noble, Fincher, Park, & Press, 2014). The steps of the mediation process are as follows (Employment Practices Solutions, 2011):

- Opening statements
- Identifying the problem
- Identifying issues and agenda setting
- Finding solutions
- Reaching agreement

Mediation can be a powerful strategy for mitigating conflict. But, sometimes, conflict is not direct or easily apprehensible. Rather, conflict and harsh behaviors may be so ingrained in a workplace that they become part of the environment in an ongoing way. Such environments are stressful and toxic and specific strategies must be used to help nurses navigate these toxic workplaces.

NAVIGATING A TOXIC WORKPLACE

A toxic workplace is one that has a negative effect on employees as well as the entire organization. This type of environment develops over time as a result of poor organizational practices, undesirable working conditions, and ineffective leadership, which results in widespread negative emotions within the workplace (Harder, Wagner, & Rash, 2014).

A toxic work environment in nursing threatens patient safety and can lead to medical errors. Some strategies to help nurses protect themselves within a toxic environment include the following (White & Schoonover-Shoffner, 2016):

- Document all work accurately and carefully
- Ask leaders to put instructions and requests in writing
- Include a third party at important meetings
- Focus on direct communication
- Avoid engaging in negative behaviors

CONCLUSION

Nurses are faced with numerous stressors within the work environment. Successfully overcoming conflict may involve the use of conflict mediation strategies or mediation from a third party. When the workplace itself is riddled with negativity, it can be considered toxic. Nurses must be aware of how to traverse a toxic work environment in order to protect themselves and maintain quality patient care.

References

Brubaker, D., Noble, C., Fincher, R., Park, S. K.-Y., & Press, S. (2014). Conflict resolution in the workplace: What will the future bring? *Conflict Resolution Quarterly*, *31*(4), 357–386. doi:10.1002/crq.21104

Dahlin, C. M., & Wittenberg, E. (2015). Communication in palliative care: An essential competency for nurses. In B. R. Ferrell, N. Coyle, & J. A. Paice (Eds.), *Oxford textbook of palliative nursing* (pp. 81–109). New York, NY: Oxford University Press.

Employment Practices Solutions. (2011). Mediation in the workplace: A proactive approach to preventing litigation and promoting a healthier work environment. Retrieved from http://www.epspros.com/NewsResources/Newsletters?find=12002

Harder, H. G., Wagner, S., & Rash, J. (2014). *Mental illness in the workplace: Psychological disability management*. New York, NY: Routledge.

Mallidi, J. (2015). How to handle conflict with poise? A fellow's perspective. *Journal of the American College of Cardiology*, *65* (1), 98–100. doi:10.1016/j.jacc.2014.11.012

Orly, S., Rivka, B., Rivka, E., & Dorit, S. E. (2012). Are cognitive–behavioral interventions effective in reducing occupational stress among nurses? *Applied Nursing Research*, *25*(3), 152–157. doi:10.1016/j.apnr.2011.01.004

Roberts, R., Grubb, P. L., & Grosch, J. W. (2012, June 25). Alleviating job stress in nurses. *Medscape*. Retrieved from www.medscape.com

Tjosvold, D., Wong, A. S. H., & Yi Feng Chen, N. (2014). Constructively managing conflicts in organizations. *Annual Review of Organizational Psychology and Organizational Behavior, 1*, 545–568. doi:10.1146/annurev-orgpsych-031413-091306

White, P. E., & Schoonover-Shoffner, K. (2016). Surviving (even thriving?) in a toxic workplace. *Journal of Christian Nursing, 33*(3), 142–149. doi:10.1097/CNJ.0000000000000289

Yamada, D. (2015). As workplace bullying enters the mainstream of American employment relations: Will law and public policy follow? *Members-only Library, 14*, 19–21.

21

Self-Care 101

To cope with the numerous pressures of nursing work, nurses must find ways to release negative emotions, deal with conflict, and promote their own well-being. This chapter discusses the ways to build resilience, cope with multiple patient losses, and employ self-care practices.

After reading this chapter, you will be able to:

- Identify ways to increase resilience
- Discuss ways to cope with multiple patient losses
- Utilize a variety of self-care techniques

RESILIENCE

Working in health care is extremely rewarding but also presents many challenges that can lead to burnout. Building resilience is critical for sustaining a lifelong, rewarding career in nursing. Resilience is a personality trait that enables one to overcome challenges and resolve negative emotions (Pettifer, 2013). Resilience does not mean that nurses must become discompassionate. Rather, it entails the ability to access deeply rooted emotional strength to be able to provide compassionate, quality care despite the sadness and grief that may ensue after the patient dies (Pettifer, 2013).

Although many studies have identified resilience as a trait specific to an individual, it is possible to build resilience over time. For example, external activities such as developing problem-solving skills and engaging in work, play, art, or exercise help to build resilience. Maintaining hope and consistently using positive coping skills can also foster resilience (Rushton, Batcheller, Schroeder, & Donohue, 2015). Hospice nurses must be especially resilient as they repeatedly encounter patient losses.

COPING WITH MULTIPLE LOSSES

One of the stressors that is unique to hospice nursing is the knowledge that most patients with whom the nurse forms a bond will die during the course of their relationship. Hospice nurses form very close bonds with patients and families because home visits may last 1 to 2 hours, several times each week. In inpatient settings, hospice nurses also become emotionally invested in managing each patient's symptoms and supporting family members through symptom crises and/or through the loss of their loved one. Even though hospice nurses are aware that their patients are terminally ill, recurrent exposure to the loss of patients is emotionally unsettling and can take a toll on nurses' well-being.

The death of a patient might be emotionally challenging, especially when the nurse is expected to move on quickly to the next patient. The burden of working in end-of-life settings includes not only the emotional toll, but also (Kent, Anderson, & Owens, 2012):

- Technological challenges
- Ethical dilemmas
- Legal issues
- Cultural considerations
- Family assessment and education
- Complex symptom management

Fast Facts in a Nutshell

Health care professionals who feel emotionally connected with a patient report many of the same grief symptoms as family members when the patient dies (Boerner, Burack, Jopp, & Mock, 2015).

Further, because hospice nurses often live in the same communities they serve, seeing family members of former patients in the community setting can cause additional stress (Pettifer, 2013). Providing such intimate and complex care for patients as they face the end of their lives requires enormous dedication and skill. However, the ability to manage such a delicate balance can be a motivating factor for hospice nurses and bolster their professional identity (Kent et al., 2012).

Even for experienced hospice nurses, cumulative losses can lead to compassion fatigue and burnout. Yet, the experienced nurse is a wealth of knowledge and a valued resource for patients and organizations. To help minimize the risk of burnout and promote career longevity, nurses must engage in numerous self-care strategies.

SELF-CARE STRATEGIES

The World Health Organization (2009) defines self-care as "a deliberate action that individuals, family members and the community should engage in to maintain good health" (p. 2). Self-care activities include:

- Eating well
- Exercising
- Obtaining outside interests
- Journaling
- Praying
- Meditating
- Using vacation time
- Massage
- Requesting a change of assignment, if needed

Although nurses understand the importance of self-care, they do not always consistently engage in these activities (Malloy, Thrane, Winston, Virani, & Kelly, 2013). Self-care is indeed an individual responsibility that all nurses must undertake. But, workplaces must also support and encourage nurses to take self-care seriously and provide opportunities for nurses to debrief after distressing events. Some ways to support the wellness of nurses in the workplace are as follows (Harris & Griffin, 2015):

- Availability of a reflection/meditation room
- Availability of employee support programs
- Support for time off through adequate staffing

- Rituals or ceremonies to recognize the patients who have died and to promote closure
- Public recognition for the work that nurses do
- Paid leave
- Assurance of a collegial atmosphere
- Zero tolerance for workplace bullying
- Encouraging personal journaling
- Rotating care of difficult patient assignments

Through initiatives that promote the well-being of nurses, organizations can help improve patient care as well as retain excellent employees. Work environments that encourage self-care also improve the health of their employees by making self-care the norm rather than the exception.

CONCLUSION

Through a combination of consistent use of self-care techniques and engaging in workplace initiatives to decrease stress and foster a positive work environment, nurses can reduce their risk of burnout and other work-related issues. Self-care helps nurses to consistently deliver quality patient care over the course of their careers.

References

Boerner, K., Burack, O. R., Jopp, D. S., & Mock, S. E. (2015). Grief after patient death: Direct care staff in nursing homes and homecare. *Journal of Pain and Symptom Management, 49*(2), 214–222. Retrieved from http://europepmc.org/articles/pmc4300283

Harris, C., & Griffin, M. T. Q. (2015). Nursing on empty: Compassion fatigue signs, symptoms, and system interventions. *Journal of Christian Nursing, 32*(2), 80–87. doi:10.1097/CNJ.0000000000000155

Kent, B., Anderson, N. E., & Owens, R. G. (2012). Nurses' early experiences with patient death: The results of an on-line survey of registered nurses in New Zealand. *International Journal of Nursing Studies, 49*, 1255–1265. doi:10.1016/j.ijnurstu.2012.04.005

Malloy, P., Thrane, S., Winston, T., Virani, R., & Kelly, K. (2013). Do nurses who care for patients in palliative and end-of-life settings perform good self-care? *Journal of Hospice & Palliative Nursing, 15*(2), 99–106. doi:10.1097/NJH.0b013e31826bef72

Pettifer, A. (2013). Resolving my own feelings after a patient has died. In J. De Souza & A. Pettifer (Eds.), *End-of-life nursing care: A guide for best practice* (pp. 186–197). New York, NY: Sage.

Rushton, C. H., Batcheller, J. Schroeder, K., & Donohue, P. (2015). Burnout and resilience among nurses practicing in high-intensity settings. *American Journal of Critical Care, 24*(5), 412–420. doi:10.4037/ajcc2015291

World Health Organization. (2009). Self-care in the context of primary health care. Retrieved from http://www.searo.who.int/entity/primary _health_care/documents/sea_hsd_320.pdf

Appendix

SAMPLE POLST FORM

		Last Name
pennsylvania DEPARTMENT OF HEALTH	**Pennsylvania Orders for Life-Sustaining Treatment (POLST)**	First/Middle Initial
		Date of Birth

FIRST follow these orders, **THEN** contact physician, certified registered nurse practitioner or physician assistant. This is an Order Sheet based on the person's medical condition and wishes at the time the orders were issued. Everyone shall be treated with dignity and respect.

A Check One	**CARDIOPULMONARY RESUSCITATION (CPR): Person has no pulse <u>and</u> is not breathing.** ☐ CPR/Attempt Resuscitation ☐ DNR/Do Not Attempt Resuscitation (Allow Natural Death) When not in cardiopulmonary arrest, follow orders in **B, C** and **D.**
B Check One	**MEDICAL INTERVENTIONS: Person has pulse <u>and/or</u> is breathing.** ☐ **COMFORT MEASURES ONLY** Use medication by any route, positioning, wound care and other measures to relieve pain and suffering. Use oxygen, oral suction and manual treatment of airway obstruction as needed for comfort. *Do not transfer to hospital for life-sustaining treatment. Transfer if comfort needs cannot be met in current location.* ☐ **LIMITED ADDITIONAL INTERVENTIONS** Includes care described above. Use medical treatment, IV fluids and cardiac monitor as indicated. Do not use intubation, advanced airway interventions, or mechanical ventilation. *Transfer to hospital if indicated. Avoid intensive care if possible.* ☐ **FULL TREATMENT** Includes care described above. Use intubation, advanced airway interventions, mechanical ventilation, and cardioversion as indicated. *Transfer to hospital if indicated. Includes intensive care.* *Additional Orders* _____

(continued)

SEND FORM WITH PERSON WHENEVER TRANSFERRED OR DISCHARGED (*continued*)

<table>
<tr>
<td rowspan="2">C
Check
One</td>
<td>ANTIBIOTICS:

☐ No antibiotics. Use other measures to relieve symptoms.
☐ Determine use or limitation of antibiotics when infection occurs, with comfort as goal.
☐ Use antibiotics if life can be prolonged.

Additional Orders</td>
<td rowspan="2">D
Check
One</td>
<td>ARTIFICIALLY ADMINIS-TERED HYDRATION / NUTRITION:
Always offer food and liquids by mouth if feasible.

☐ No hydration and artificial nutrition by tube.
☐ Trial period of artificial hydration and nutrition by tube.
☐ Long-term artificial hydration and nutrition by tube.

Additional Orders</td>
</tr>
</table>

<table>
<tr>
<td rowspan="6">E
Check
One</td>
<td colspan="3">SUMMARY OF GOALS, MEDICAL CONDITION AND SIGNATURES:</td>
</tr>
<tr>
<td colspan="2">Discussed with
☐ Patient
☐ Parent of Minor
☐ Health Care Agent
☐ Health Care Representative
☐ Court-Appointed Guardian
☐ Other:</td>
<td>Patient Goals/Medical Condition:</td>
</tr>
<tr>
<td colspan="3">By signing this form, I acknowledge that this request regarding resuscitative measures is consistent with the known desires of, and in the best interest of, the individual who is the subject of the form.</td>
</tr>
<tr>
<td colspan="2">Physician/PA/CRNP Printed Name:</td>
<td>Physician/PA/CRNP Phone Number</td>
</tr>
<tr>
<td colspan="2">Physician/PA/CRNP Signature (Required):</td>
<td>DATE</td>
</tr>
<tr>
<td colspan="3">Signature of Patient or Surrogate</td>
</tr>
</table>

Signature (required)	Name (print)	Relationship (write "self" if patient)

(*continued*)

SEND FORM WITH PERSON WHENEVER TRANSFERRED OR DISCHARGED (continued)

Other Contact Information

Surrogate	Relationship	Phone Number	
Health Care Professional Preparing Form	Preparer Title	Phone Number	Date Prepared

Directions for Health care Professionals

Any individual for whom a Pennsylvania Order for Life-Sustaining Treatment form is completed should ideally have an advance health care directive that provides instructions for the individual's health care and appoints an agent to make medical decisions whenever the patient is unable to make or communicate a health care decision. If the patient wants a DNR Order issued in section "A", the physician/PA/CRNP should discuss the issuance of an Out-of-Hospital DNR order, if the individual is eligible, to assure that an EMS provider can honor his/her wishes. Contact the Pennsylvania Department of Aging for information about sample forms for advance health care directives. Contact the Pennsylvania Department of Health, Bureau of EMS, for information about Out-of Hospital Do-Not-Resuscitate orders, bracelets and necklaces. POLST forms may be obtained online from the Pennsylvania Department of Health. www.health.state.pa.us

Completing POLST

Must be completed by a health care professional based on patient preferences and medical indications or decisions by the patient or a surrogate. This document refers to the person for whom the orders are issued as the "individual" or "patient" and refers to any other person authorized to make health care decisions for the patient covered by this document as the "surrogate."

At the time a POLST is completed, any current advance directive, if available, must be reviewed.

Must be signed by a physician/PA/CRNP and patient/surrogate to be valid. Verbal orders are acceptable with follow-up signature by physician/PA/CRNP and patient/surrogate to be valid. Verbal orders are acceptable with follow-up signature by physician/PA/CRNP in accordance with facility/community policy. A person designated by the patient or surrogate may document the patient's agreement. Use of original form is strongly encouraged. Photocopies and Faxes of signed POLST forms should be respected where necessary.

(continued)

SEND FORM WITH PERSON WHENEVER TRANSFERRED OR DISCHARGED (continued)

Using POLST

If a person's condition changes and time permits, the patient or surrogate must be contacted to assure that the POLST is updated as appropriate.

If any section is not completed, then the health care provider should follow other appropriate methods to determine treatment.

An automated external defibrillator (AED) should not be used on a person who has chosen "Do Not Attempt Resuscitation"

Oral fluids and nutrition must always be offered if medically feasible.

When comfort cannot be achieved in the current setting, the person, including someone with "comfort measures only," should be transferred to a setting able to provide comfort (e.g., treatment of a hip fracture).

A person who chooses either "comfort measures only" or "limited additional interventions" may not require transfer or referral to a facility with a higher level of care.

An IV medication to enhance comfort may be appropriate for a person who has chosen "Comfort Measures Only."

Treatment of dehydration is a measure which may prolong life. A person who desires IV fluids should indicate "Limited Additional Interventions" or "Full Treatment."

A patient with or without capacity or the surrogate who gave consent to this order or who is otherwise specifically authorized to do so, can revoke consent to any part of this order providing for the withholding or withdrawal of life-sustaining treatment, at any time, and request alternative treatment.

Review

This form should be reviewed periodically (consider at least annually) and a new form completed if necessary when:
(1) The person is transferred from one care setting or care level to another, or
(2) There is a substantial change in the person's health status, or
(3) The person's treatment preferences change.

Revoking POLST

If the POLST becomes invalid or is replaced by an updated version, draw a line through sections A through E of the invalid POLST, write "VOID" in large letters across the form, and sign and date the form.

Source: Pennsylvania Department of Health (2010). Pennsylvania orders for life-sustaining treatment (POLST). Retrieved from http://www.upmc.com/Services/AgingInstitute/partnerships-and-collaborations/Documents/POLST-Form.pdf

CRNP, certified registered nurse practitioner; EMS, emergency medical services; IV, intravenous; PA, physician assistant.

FAST SCALE

FAST SCALE ADMINISTRATION

The FAST scale is a functional scale designed to evaluate patients at the more moderate-severe stages of dementia when the Mini-Mental Status Examination (MMSE) no longer can reflect changes in a meaningful clinical way. In the early stages the patient may be able to participate in the FAST administration but usually the information should be collected from a caregiver or, in the case of nursing home care, the nursing home staff.

The FAST scale has seven stages:
1. **which is normal adult**
2. **which is normal older adult**
3. **which is early dementia**
4. **which is mild dementia**
5. **which is moderate dementia**
6. **which is moderately severe dementia**
7. **which is severe dementia**

FAST Functional Milestones

FAST stage 1 is the normal adult with no cognitive decline. FAST stage 2 is the normal older adult with very mild memory loss. Stage 3 is early dementia. Here memory loss becomes apparent to coworkers and family. Patients may be unable to remember names of persons just introduced to them. Stage 4 is mild dementia. Persons in this stage may have difficulty with finances, counting money, and travel to new locations. Memory loss increases. The person's knowledge of current and recent events decreases. Stage 5 is moderate dementia. In this stage, the person needs more help to survive. He or she does not need assistance with toileting or eating, but does need help choosing clothing. The person displays increased difficulty with serial subtraction. Patients may not know the date and year or where they live. However, they do know who they are and the names of their family and friends. Stage 6 is moderately severe dementia. The person may begin to forget the names of family members or friends. The person requires more assistance with activities of daily living, such as bathing, toileting, and eating. Patients in this stage may develop delusions, hallucinations, or obsessions. Patients show increased anxiety and may become violent. The person in this stage begins to sleep during the day and stay awake at night. Stage 6 is severe dementia. In this stage, all speech is lost. Patients lose urinary and bowel control. They lose the ability to walk. Most become bedridden and die of sepsis or pneumonia.

Functional Assessment Staging of Alzheimer's Disease. (FAST)©

STAGE	SKILL LEVEL
1.	No difficulties, either subjectively or objectively.
2.	Complains of forgetting location of objects. Subjective word finding difficulties.
3.	Decreased job function evident to co-workers; difficulty in traveling to new locations. Decreased organizational capacity.*
4.	Decreased ability to perform complex tasks (e.g., planning dinner for guests), handling personal finances (forgetting to pay bills), difficulty marketing, etc.
5.	Requires assistance in choosing proper clothing to wear for day, season, occasion.
6a.	Difficulty putting clothing on properly without assistance.
b.	Unable to bathe properly (e.g., difficulty adjusting bath water temperature) occasionally or more frequently over the past weeks.*
c.	Inability to handle mechanics of toileting (e.g., forgets to flush the toilet, does not wipe properly or properly dispose of toilet tissue) occasionally or more frequently over the past weeks.*
d.	Urinary incontinence, occasional or more frequent.
e.	Fecal incontinence (occasional or more frequently over the past week).
7a.	Ability to speak limited to approximately a half dozen different words or fewer, in the course of an average day or in the course of an intensive interview.
b.	Speech ability limited to the use of a single intelligible word in an average day or in the course of an interview (the person may repeat the word over and over).
c.	Ambulatory ability lost (cannot walk without personal assistance).
d.	Ability to sit up without assistance lost (e.g., the individual will fall over if there are no lateral rests [arms] on the chair).
e.	Loss of the ability to smile.

STAGE • • _____

*Scored primarily on the basis of information obtained from a knowledgeable informant and/or caregiver.

©1984 by Barry Reisberg, M.D. All rights reserved. Reisberg, B. Functional Assessment Staging (FAST). Psychopharmacology Bulletin. 1988:24: 653–659.

KARNOFSKY SCALE

The Karnofsky Performance Scale

The Karnofsky scale was devised by two American doctors in the 1940s (David Karnofsky and Joseph Burchenal) as an attempt to try to measure the more "subjective" side of the outcome of cancer treatment.

In fact the scale relates purely to physical ability and covers 11 points, from normal health to death, each scored as a percentage. The scale is:

Karnofsky Score (KS)	Definition
100	Normal; no complaints; no evidence of disease
90	Able to carry on normal activity; minor signs or symptoms of disease
80	Normal activity with effort; some sign or symptoms of disease
70	Cares for self; unable to carry on normal activity or do active work
60	Requires occasional assistance, but is able to care for most personal needs
50	Requires considerable assistance and frequent medical care
40	Disabled; requires special care and assistance
30	Severely disabled; hospitalization is indicated, although death not imminent
20	Very sick; hospitalization necessary; active support treatment is necessary
10	Moribund; fatal processes progressing rapidly
0	Dead

Source: Karnofsky, D. A., & Burchenal, J. H. (1949). The clinical evaluation of chemotherapeutic agents in cancer. In C. M. MacLeod (Ed.), *Evaluation of chemotherapeutic agents.* New York, NY: Columbia University Press.

PALLIATIVE PERFORMANCE SCALE (PPS-2)

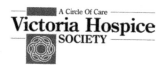

A Circle Of Care

Victoria Hospice
SOCIETY

Palliative Performance Scale (Ppsv-2)

version 2

PPS Level	Ambulation	Activity & Evidence of Disease	Self-care	Intake	Conscious Level
100%	Full	Normal activity & work No evidence of disease	Full	Normal	Full
90%	Full	Normal activity & work Some evidence of disease	Full	Normal	Full
80%	Full	Normal activity *with* effort Some evidence of disease	Full	Normal or reduced	Full
70%	Reduced	Unable normal job/work Significant disease	Full	Normal or reduced	Full
60%	Reduced	Unable hobby/house work Significant disease	Occasional assistance necessary	Normal or reduced	Full or Confusion
50%	Mainly Sit/Lie	Unable to do any work Extensive disease	Considerable assistance required	Normal or reduced	Full or Confusion
40%	Mainly in Bed	Unable to do most activity Extensive disease	Mainly assistance	Normal or reduced	Full or Drowsy +/− Confusion
30%	Totally Bed Bound	Unable to do any activity Extensive disease	Total Care	Normal or reduced	Full or Drowsy +/− Confusion
20%	Totally Bed Bound	Unable to do any activity Extensive disease	Total Care	Minimal to sips	Full or Drowsy +/− Confusion
10%	Totally Bed Bound	Unable to do any activity Extensive disease	Total Care	Mouth care only	Drowsy or Coma +/− Confusion
0%	Death	-	-	-	-

Instructions for Use of PPS (see also definition of terms)

1. PPS scores are determined by reading horizontally at each level to find a "best fit" for the patient which is then assigned as the PPS% score.

2. Begin at the left column and read downwards until the appropriate ambulation level is reached, then read across to the next column and downwards again until the activity/evidence of disease is located. These steps are repeated until all five columns are covered before assigning the actual PPS for that patient. In this way, "leftward" columns (columns to the left of any specific column) are "stronger" determinants and generally take precedence over others.

   Example 1: A patient who spends the majority of the day sitting or lying down due to fatigue from advanced disease and requires considerable assistance to walk even for short distances but who is otherwise fully conscious level with good intake would be scored at PPS 50%.

   Example 2: A patient who has become paralyzed and quadriplegic requiring total care would be PPS 30%. Although this patient may be placed in a wheelchair (and perhaps seem initially to be at 50%), the score is 30% because he or she would be otherwise totally bed bound due to the disease or complication if it were not for caregivers providing total care including lift/transfer. The patient may have normal intake and full conscious level.

   Example 3: However, if the patient in example 2 was paraplegic and bed bound but still able to do some self-care such as feed him or herself, then the PPS would be higher at 40% or 50% since he or she is not "total care."

3. PPS scores are in 10% increments only. Sometimes, there are several columns easily placed at one level but one or two that seem better at a higher or lower level. One then needs to make a "best fit" decision. Choosing a "half-fit" value of PPS 45%, for example, is not correct. The combination of clinical judgment and "leftward precedence" is used to determine whether 40% or 50% is the more accurate score for that patient.

4. PPS may be used for several purposes. First, it is an excellent communication tool for quickly describing a patient's current functional level. Second, it may have value in criteria for workload assessment or other measurements and comparisons. Finally, it appears to have prognostic value.

Definition of Terms for PPS

As noted below, some of the terms have similar meanings with the differences being more readily apparent as one reads horizontally across each row to find an overall "best fit" using all five columns.

1. Ambulation

The items "**mainly sit/lie**," "**mainly in bed**," and "**totally bed bound**" are clearly similar. The subtle differences are related to items in the self-care column. For example, "totally bed bound" at PPS 30% is due to either profound weakness or paralysis such that the patient not only can't get out of bed but is also unable to do any self-care. The difference between "sit/lie" and "bed" is proportionate to the amount of time the patient is able to sit up versus the need to lie down.

"**Reduced ambulation**" is located at the PPS 70% and PPS 60% level. By using the adjacent column, the reduction of ambulation is tied to inability to carry out the person's normal job, work occupation or some hobbies or housework activities. The person is still able to walk and transfer on his or her own but at PPS 60% needs occasional assistance.

2. Activity & Extent of disease

"**Some**," "**significant**," and "**extensive**" disease refer to physical and investigative evidence that shows degrees of progression. For example in breast cancer, a local recurrence would imply "some" disease, one or two metastases in the lung or bone would imply "significant" disease, whereas multiple metastases in lung, bone, liver, brain, hypercalcemia or other major complications would be "extensive" disease. The extent may also refer to progression of disease despite active treatments. Using PPS in AIDS, "some" may mean the shift from HIV to AIDS, "significant" implies progression in physical decline, new or difficult symptoms and laboratory findings with low counts. "Extensive" refers to one or more serious complications with or without continuation of active antiretrovirals, antibiotics, and so forth.

The above extent of disease is also judged in context with the ability to maintain one's work and hobbies or activities. Decline in activity may mean the person still plays golf but reduces from playing 18 holes to 9 holes, or just a par 3, or to backyard putting. People who enjoy walking will gradually reduce the distance covered, although they may continue trying, sometimes even close to death (e.g., trying to walk the halls).

3. Self-Care

"**Occasional assistance**" means that most of the time patients are able to transfer out of bed, walk, wash, toilet and eat by their own means, but that on occasion (perhaps once daily or a few times weekly) they require minor assistance.

"**Considerable assistance**" means that regularly every day the patient needs help, usually by one person, to do some of the activities noted above. For example, the person needs help to get to the bathroom but is then able to brush his or her teeth or wash at least hands and face. Food will often need to be cut into edible sizes but the patient is then able to eat of his or her own accord.

"**Mainly assistance**" is a further extension of "considerable." Using the above example, the patient now needs help getting up but also needs assistance washing his face and shaving, but can usually eat with minimal or no help. This may fluctuate according to fatigue during the day.

"**Total care**" means that the patient is completely unable to eat without help, toilet or do any self-care. Depending on the clinical situation, the patient may or may not be able to chew and swallow food once prepared and fed to him or her.

4. Intake

Changes in intake are quite obvious with "**normal intake**" referring to the person's usual eating habits while healthy.

"**Reduced**" means any reduction from that and is highly variable according to the unique individual circumstances.

"**Minimal**" refers to very small amounts, usually pureed or liquid, which are well below nutritional sustenance.

5. Conscious Level

"**Full consciousness**" implies full alertness and orientation with good cognitive abilities in various domains of thinking, memory, and so forth. "**Confusion**" is used to denote presence of either delirium or dementia and is a reduced level of consciousness. It may be mild, moderate or severe with multiple possible etiologies. "**Drowsiness**" implies either fatigue, drug side effects, delirium or closeness to death and is sometimes included in the term "stupor." "**Coma**" in this context is the absence of response to verbal or physical stimuli; some reflexes may or may not remain. The depth of coma may fluctuate throughout a 24-hour period.

Index